MONSEN AND BAER

The Beauty of Perfume

Perfume Bottle Auction VI

May 11, 1996.

Auction:
Hyatt Regency Hotel
San Francisco Airport
1333 Bayshore Hwy.
Burlingame, California

Auctioneer: Michael DeFina

**Auction Preview: All lots will be available for viewing
and inspection from 10:00 AM to 5:00 PM on Saturday, May 11, 1996.
Sale will begin at 5:00 PM, May 11, 1996.**

Monsen and Baer
Box 529
Vienna, VA 22183 USA
(703) 938-2129
Fax (703) 242-1357

ISBN #0-9636102-4-4

The Beauty of Perfume

Table of Contents

Preface

To our fellow collectors in this country and abroad, greetings and good wishes! This is the sixth fully catalogued auction of perfume bottles to be held in the United States--the only auction of its kind devoted solely to perfume bottles and memorabilia of the fragrance industry--and this auction serves to support the International Perfume Bottle Association in that it is held during the annual IPBA Convention, and that a portion of the proceeds of the auction will be donated to that organization. If you are a serious collector of perfume bottles, you should become a member of the IPBA, the International Perfume Bottle Association. The IPBA publishes a wonderful Quarterly, a Membership Directory, and organizes an outstanding annual Convention. We will happily send membership information to all who request it.

This year, we have produced a book, *The Beauty of Perfume*, in hard cover, containing descriptions of all the lots in the auction. Our catalogue began as a listing of lots for the auction, but it has developed into something that is much more than that. The photographs and descriptions of lots serve the obvious and primary function of information for the auction sale, but beyond that, they also have an archival function that collectors in the United States and abroad are coming to value highly. Our overall goal is to provide the collector with a resource of documentation that can be used over and over again. The new book format provides a more durable object for collectors to use and re-use. We have produced this book without any additional cost passed on to those who purchase it. The goal here goes beyond merely selling perfume bottles, though of course we wish to do that and to do it well. In a very real sense, we want to produce for collectors something that we, as collectors ourselves, would value and find useful. Our sincere wish is that other collectors use it, learn from it, and enjoy it.

The article section of this book further expands its documentation and research goals, and allows this information to be shared among our many international readers. To aid in the expansion and diffusion of knowledge about perfume bottles, we have again prevailed upon fellow collectors and dealers to share their invaluable knowledge on a variety of subjects. As we did last year, we also include translations of these articles in French and German. We are indebted to Peter Dechent, Thomas Cory, Christiane Angeli, and Thomas Higonnet for this work. The article section allows authors to discuss a specific topic in great detail, and allows each author to reach a wide audience, in the USA and abroad. *We produce this section as a service to this wonderful hobby: What we have said in the past bears repeating here: Knowledge–and the sharing of it– enhances our pleasure in collecting.*

We are quite convinced that collectors of the rather near future will look back longingly and wistfully upon this sale and will recognize that it was in fact an opportunity to acquire incredibly desirable perfume bottles at advantageous prices. Our hope is that each collector of today will also recognize this opportunity to acquire a wonderful perfume bottle for their collection.

We would like to encourage other collectors to research and to write about the subject of perfume bottles. If you have an advanced collection of a particular type of perfume bottle, you may well have the basis for an article. There are many topics of great interest but about which there is practically no published information, and the only possible source of such information may be in the collections which have been assembled by individual collectors.

If you have a truly wonderful perfume bottle that you would consider selling, then our 1997 auction, to be held near Washington, D. C., may be the perfect venue to do so. For those who would like to consign bottles for the 1997 auction, please contact us soon after this sale. Consignment details will be sent to those who request this information.

We particularly thank the consignors and the contributors of articles to this catalogue.

Books Available from:

Monsen and Baer
Box 529
Vienna, VA 22183 USA

Baccarat Les Flacons à Parfum/The Perfume Bottles [Cie. des Cristalleries de Baccarat]
@ $79.95 + $7 shipping.§
Made in Czechoslovakia, Book 2 [R. Forsythe] @ $29.95 + $5 shipping.¶
Avon Bottle Collector's Encyclopedia (13th Edition) [B. Hastin] @ $19.95 + $7 shipping.§
Commercial Perfume Bottles [J. Jones-North] @ $69.95 + $7 shipping.§
Guerlain: A Century of Minis: 1895-1995, by Michèle Atlas and Alain Monniot. Milan
Editions 160 pp, text in English and French @ $60 + $7 shipping.
Lalique Perfume Bottles [M. L. and G. Utt and P. Bayer] @ $35 + $7 shipping.§

We can ship the above books to Europe, but the cost is as follows: *§These books can be shipped to Europe for an additional $27 each.* *¶These books can be shipped to Europe for an additional $16 each.*

The following auction catalogues are also available, all postpaid and with Prices Realized:
Monsen and Baer Perfume Bottle Auction I,
    Chicago, April 6, 1991 @ $18.00. ($25 for International shipment).
Monsen and Baer Perfume Bottle Auction II,
    Atlanta, May 16, 1992 @ $25.00. ($30 for International shipment).
Monsen and Baer Perfume Bottle Auction III,
    Dallas, May 1, 1993 @$28.00. ($35 for International shipment).
Monsen and Baer Perfume Bottle Auction IV,
    Washington, D. C., May 14, 1994 @ $29.00. ($35 for International shipment).
Monsen and Baer Perfume Bottle Auction V,
    Chicago, Illinois, May 6, 1995 @ $35.00. ($40 for International shipment).
The Beauty of Perfume, Monsen and Baer Perfume Bottle Auction VI,
    San Francisco, California, May 11, 1996. ($45 for International shipment.)

The Conditions of Sale
All lots sold in this auction are subject to the following conditions: please read carefully.

Terms of Sale. All lots will be sold, in the numerical sequence of this catalogue, to the highest bidder as determined by the auctioneer. In the case of disputed bids, the auctioneer shall have the sole discretion of determining the purchaser, and may elect to reoffer the lot for sale. We will accept cash, travelers checks, or personal checks with acceptable identification or if the buyer is known to us; we reserve the right in some cases to ship the lot to the purchaser after their check has cleared.

Sales Tax. All lots are subject to 8.25% California state sales tax unless a valid tax exemption form has been filed with us.

Absentee Bids. A form for absentee bids is available. We will be happy to execute your bid for you as if you were present at the auction. When you do this, it does not mean that the bidding will commence with your bid, it simply means that we will not bid for you above the amount you indicate. It is advantageous to place these absentee bids as early as possible. In the case of identical bids, the bid from the floor will take precedence; for identical absentee bids, the earlier-dated bid will take precedence. We are unable to accept telephone bids. Please read shipping information below.

Bidding Increments. Bidding increments are totally at the discretion of the auctioneer. However, the following increments are typically used: under $50, increments of $5; $50-$300, increments of $10; $300-$500, increments of $25; $500-$1,000, increments of $50; $1,000-$3,000, increments of $100; $3,000-$5,000, increments of $250; $5,000-$10,000, increments of $500; above $10,000, increments of $1,000.

Shipping. We offer the possibility of shipping your purchases anywhere. For the United States and Canada, the flat charge for this service is $15 per lot for lots whose sale price is less than $1000; the charges will be higher for the lots valued over $1000 due to insurance charges. Lots which consist of large items can be shipped, with actual shipping charges to be paid by the purchaser.

Shipping purchases to Europe is also possible. **There is a charge for this service of $15 for each lot purchased, plus the actual cost of the shipping.** Absentee bidders will be sent an invoice for the shipping charges and balance due; we offer the convenience of accepting payment in all major European currencies. We normally use United Parcel Service or DHL to ship to Europe. This service is highly reliable and extremely rapid. However, please note that the minimum charge for a small parcel sent by UPS to Europe is $75. Parcels consisting of several lots may cost twice that amount. If the purchaser specifically requests it, we can also ship via the Postal Service. Lots which are shipped outside the United States are subject to customs duties in the destination country. It is the responsibility of the purchaser to determine the amount of these duties and to pay them in full.

Price Estimates and Reserves. Some lots, typically those with a value in excess of one thousand dollars, are offered for sale with a "reserve price." The reserve is a confidential minimum price below which the lot will not be sold. The reserve price for any lot in this sale is usually well below the low estimate and is never allowed to be higher than the estimates. The estimates are merely a range within which we believe the lot may find a buyer, but of course many lots may be sold at prices well below or well above these estimates, depending on the wishes of the bidders.

Buyer's Premium. A buyer's premium of 10% will be added to the hammer price of all lots, to be paid by the buyer as a part of the purchase price.

Condition of Lots. While we attempt to describe the condition of each lot as accurately as possible, as in all auctions, the lots here are sold "as is." Notes on the salient condition of lots are provided in parentheses in the lot description, for example: [label absent], [chip to stopper], etc. However, many factors relating to condition cannot be adequately described in the short captions of this catalogue. Very many perfume bottles have exceedingly tiny chips around the opening where the stopper enters the bottle. Sometimes these may also be found on the tongue of the stopper or on the base of the bottle. The boxes and labels of commercial bottles may all show varying signs of usage and age, such as discoloration and fraying. All bottles, and especially commercial ones, may contain perfume residue and other internal stains. Not all stoppers fit into the bottle with perfect snugness and symmetry, especially those of Czechoslovakian manufacture. Therefore, bidders should inspect each lot they wish to bid on. We would also be happy to discuss the condition of any lot prior to the sale. Measurements given in this catalogue are in inches and centimeters, rounded in most cases to the nearest quarter inch or half-centimeter. Unless stated otherwise, the bottles are empty of perfume.

In cases where glass by a particular maker is described as unsigned, the catalogue can only provide a reasonable surmise, not a guarantee, as to the maker. Many of the early French glass makers produced glass of similar quality and design. In these cases, the buyer should consult the available reference works and thereafter make their own determination. The glass made by Lalique is all grouped together under the generic heading "French Glass Artisans...R. Lalique"; this

includes bottles designed after René Lalique's death by Marc and Marie Claude Lalique. Following the convention used in Utt (1990), perfume bottles produced for sale by R. Lalique & Cie. are referred to as Maison Lalique.

Reference numbers are provided for Lalique, Baccarat, and in many cases for Czech glass, as described in Utt (1990), Compagnie des Cristalleries de Baccarat (1986), North (1990), and Forsythe I & II (1982 & 1993). These reference numbers are also used in the article section of the catalogue.

Consignments. We will be accepting consignments for a seventh auction, and we are particularly in search of fine perfume bottles. Our rates of consignment are very competitive with other auctions, and we can offer exposure of your bottles to a specialized buying audience. We guarantee confidentiality. We also purchase individual bottles or entire collections out-right, if that avenue of sale is preferred. Contact us and we would be happy to discuss these terms with you. We are especially interested in perfume bottles of high quality, not broken or damaged pieces. Please bear in mind that consignments for the 1997 auction must be completed by December 31, 1996 to allow sufficient time for the preparation of the catalogue.

References:

Ball, J. D. and Torem, D. H. *Commercial Fragrance Bottles*. Atglen, Pennsylvania: Schiffer Publishing Co., 1993.

Barille, Elisabeth. *Coty*. Paris: Editions Assouline, 1995.

Berger, C. & D. *Tous les Parfums du Monde*. Toulouse: Editions Milan, 1995.

Bonduelle, J. P. et Lancry, J. M. *Flacons à Parfums Catalogues pour les Ventes aux Enchères Publiques*: March 31, 1990; March 24, 1991; June 16, 1991; October 24, 1991; June 21, 1992; May 16, 1993; November 21, 1993; March 27, 1994; November 20, 1994; June 18, 1995; December 3, 1995; expert: J.-M. Martin-Hattemberg.

Bohnams *Scent Bottle and Lalique auction catalogues*: November 29, 1989; October 18, 1990; November 21, 1990; April 24, 1991; October 24, 1991; October 28, 1991; April 28, 1992; October 29, 1992; April 7, 1993; June 28, 1993; October 20, 1993; expert: Juliette Bogaers.

Chassaing, Rivet, Fournié. *Flacons à Parfums Catalogue pour la Vente aux Enchères Publiques*: June 27, 1994, Toulouse, France; expert: Geneviève Fontan.

Cohet et Feraud *Floréal Perfume Bottle Auction Catalogue*, Toulouse, France, April 15-16, 1995; November 4, 1995; expert: Flora Entajan.

Colard, Grégoire. *[Caron] The Secret Charm of a Perfumed House*. Paris: J. C. Lattès, 1984.

Compagnie des Cristalleries de Baccarat. *Baccarat Les Flacons à Parfum/The Perfume Bottles*. Paris: Henri Addor & Associés, 1986.

Courset, J-M. *5000 Miniatures de Parfum*. Toulouse: Editions Milan, 1995.

Coutau-Bégarie, O. *Flacons à Parfums Catalogues pour les Ventes aux Enchères Publiques*: December 6, 1993; October 24, 1994; June 12, 1995; November 27, 1995; expert: Régine de Robien.

Duval, René. *Parfums de Volnay*. Catalogue of the Company, 1928.

Drouot-Richelieu, Neret-Minet, Coutau-Begarie. *Flacons à Parfums Catalogues pour les Ventes aux Enchères Publiques*: June 23, 1986; April 2, 1987; November 4, 1987; April 13, 1988; November 7, 1988; May 20, 1989; November 13, 1989; May 21, 1990; November 24, 1990; April 8, 1991; May 27, 1991; November 15, 1991; December 14, 1992; expert: Régine de Robien.

Drouot-Richelieu, Neret-Minet. *Flacons à Parfums Catalogue pour la Vente aux Enchères Publiques*: December 14, 1992; expert: J.-M. Martin-Hattemberg.

Drouot-Richelieu, Millon & Robert. *Flacons à Parfums: Catalogue pour la Vente aux Enchères Publiques*: December 6, 1991; expert: Régine de Robien.

Duchesne, Clarence, ed. *La Mémoire des Parfums*, Numeros 1-11. Paris, 1988-1991.

Fellous, Colette. *Guerlain*. Paris: Denoël, 1987.

Fleck, F. *Flacons à Parfum, Catalogue* for the Perfume Bottle Auction, March 12, 1994; expert: Anne Meter-Seguin.

Fontan, Geneviève, and Barnouin, Nathalie. *L'Argus des Echantillons de Parfum*. Toulouse: Editions Milan, 1992.

Fontan, Geneviève, and Barnouin, Nathalie. *La Cote Internationale des Echantillons de Parfum, 1995-1996. Les Echantillons Anciens*. Toulouse: 813 Edition, 1994.

Fontan, Geneviève, and Barnouin, Nathalie. *La Cote Internationale des Echantillons de Parfums Modernes*. Toulouse: 813 Edition, 1995.

Forsythe, Ruth. *Made in Czechoslovakia*. Marietta, Ohio: Richardson Printing Co., 1982; *Made in Czechoslovakia, Book 2*. Marietta Ohio: Richardson Printing Co., 1993.

Frankl, Beatrice. *Parfum-Flacons*. Augsburg: Battenberg Verlag, 1994.

Ghozland, F. *Perfume Fantasies*. Toulouse: Editions Milan, 1987.

Guinn, Hugh D. *The Glass of René Lalique at Auction*. Tulsa, Oklahoma: Guindex Publications, 1992.

Hymne au Parfum: Catalogue de l'exposition, 1990-1991. Paris: Comité Français du Parfum, 1991.

Kaufman, William I. *Perfume*. New York: E. P. Dutton & Co., 1974.

E. H. Killian. *Perfume Bottles Remembered*. Traverse City, Michigan: E. Killian, 1989.

René Lalique and Cristal Lalique Perfume Bottles (The Weinstein Collection). New York: Christie's/Lalique Society of America, 1993.

René Lalique et Cie. *Lalique Glass: The Complete Illustrated Catalogue for 1932*. Reprinted by The Corning Museum of Glass, Corning, New York. New York: Dover Publications, 1981.

Lefkowith, Christie Mayer. *The Art of Perfume*. New York: Thames and Hudson, 1994.

Le Louvre des Antiquaires. *Autour du Parfum du XVIe au XIXe Siècle*. Paris: Le Louvre des Antiquaires, 1985.

Marcilhac, Félix. *R. Lalique: Catalogue Raisonné de l'Oeuvre de Verre*. Paris: Editions de l'Amateur, 1989.

Martin, Hazel. *Figural Perfume and Scent Bottles*. Lancaster, CA: Hazel Martin, 1982.

Matthews, Leslie G. *The Antiques of Perfume*. London: G. Bell & Sons, 1973.

Neret-Minet. *Flacons à Parfums Catalogue pour les Ventes aux Enchères Publiques*, November 14, 1991; expert: Elisabeth Danenberg.

North, Jacquelyne. *Commercial Perfume Bottles*. West Chester, Pennsylvania: Schiffer Publishing Co, 1987.

North, Jacquelyne. *Czechoslovakian Perfume Bottles and Boudoir Accessories*. Marietta, Ohio: Antique Publications, 1990.

North, Jacquelyne. *Perfume, Cologne, and Scent Bottles*. West Chester, Pennsylvania: Schiffer Publishing Co, 1986.

Parfum, Art, et Valeur. Catalogue de Vente, November 15, 1995. Expert: Geneviève Fontan.

La Quinzaine du Parfum *Perfume Bottle Auction Catalogue* for the sale of October 21, 1994; expert: Creezy Courtoy. Brussels, Belgium.

Restrepo, Federico. *Le Livre d'Heures des Flacons et des Rêves*. Toulouse: Editions Milan, 1995.

Sloan, Jean. *Perfume and Scent Bottle Collecting*. Lombard, Illinois: Wallace-Homestead Co., 1986.

Utt, Mary Lou and Glenn. *Lalique Perfume Bottles*. New York: Crown Publishers, 1990.

D. Watine-Arnault. *Flacons à Parfums Christian Dior: Catalogue pour la Vente aux Enchères Publiques*: April 12, 1992; expert: Régine de Robien.

Whitmyer, M. & K. *Bedroom and Bathroom Glassware of the Depression Years*. Paducah, Kentucky: Collector Books, 1990.

MINIATURES
SAMPLES
FLACONS DE SAC
FIRST SIZES
NOVELTIES

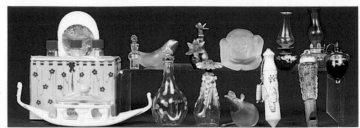

Lot #1. Perfumer's Workshop *Tea Rose;* bottle with pink cap in a plastic gondola; Avon mouse and a bird; two miniature lamp perfumes; Fabergé *Flambeau* whistle; glass vial in a celluloid case; Plantation Garden hatpin vial; four small glass bottles, some decorated with shells; *Milady's Vanity* set of three glass vials in a dresser-box. 14 items. Est. $70.00-$140.00.

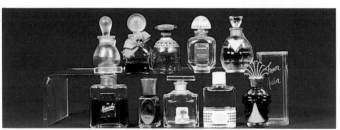

Lot #2. Avon *Unforgettable* with metal stopper; Kay Daumit *Forever Amber* with gold fan stopper and lucite case; Halston [?] with frosted teardrop stopper; Barroché *Prologue;* Vigny *Beau Catcher;* Langlois *Cara Nome;* De Rauch *Vacarme; Le Petite Tiffany* with brass cap; Grès *Cabochard;* Dior *Diorissimo* Eau de Toilette. Ten items. Est. $75.00-$125.00.

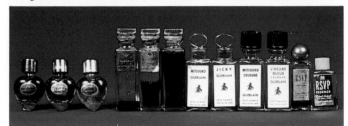

Lot #3. Lot of 12 minis: Guerlain *Mitsouko, L'Heure Bleue* testers with black caps, *Jicky, Mitsouko* testers with glass stoppers; Lanselle *Coeur, Carreau,* one without label, glass testers; Hudnut *RSVP* [two different]; Avon *Unforgettable, Cotillion, Here's My Heart* heart-shaped glass bottles with brass caps. Twelve miniatures. Est. $100.00-$200.00.

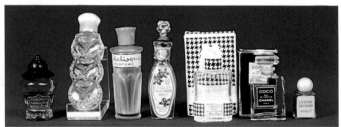

Lot #4. Lot of 7 miniatures: Ricci *Coeur Joie,* bottle with three hearts; Lelong *Indiscret;* Duchess of Paris *Infatuation;* Hanson Jenks *Violet;* Dior *Miss Dior* with box [box lid torn]; Rosenstein *Odalisque;* Chanel *Coco* with box. Seven items. Est. $100.00-$150.00.

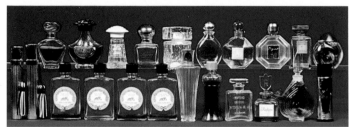

Lot #5. Lot of 22 miniatures: Borghese *Il Bacio;* Boucheron; D'Orsay glass mini [rubbed label]; Duchess of Paris *Gardenia;* Duchess of York *All of Me;* Guerlain *Shalimar* [2 different], *Chamade;* Herb Farm *Royal Purple, Night Scented Stock, White Phlox, Green Moss;* Houbigant *Essence Rare;* Lanvin *Crescendo;* Ralph Lauren *Orgeuil;* Lelong *Orgeuil;* Matchabelli *Abano* oil; Millot *Crêpe de Chine* glass tester, 2 Millot tasseled brass vials; Pucci *Vivara* glass tester; Raphael *Réplique.* 22 items. Est. $115.00-$230.00.

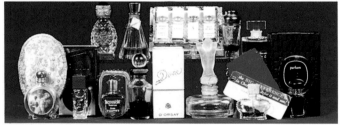

Lot #6. D'Albret *Ecusson* in its box, Dainty Dabs *The Woman I Love;* Desprez *Bal à Versailles* in its pouch; d'Orsay *Intoxication* and *Divine,* in its blue box; Fragonard *Moment Volé, 5, Belle de Nuit, Xmas* clear glass bottles with white caps, white labels, in their box printed with black lace; Gourielli *Five O'Clock* cocktail shaker; Guerlain *Nahema* in its box; *Isadora;* Lanvin *Via* in its box; Lauder *White Linen;* Matchabelli *Beloved* in its red pouch with 1956 Chevrolet tag. 12 items, 15 bottles. Est. $200.00-$300.00.

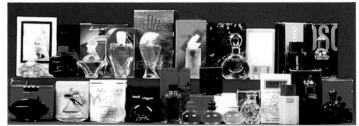

Lot #7. Collectors lot of 22 boxed miniatures: H. Alpert *Listen; Animale;* Azzaro *9;* Bill Blass *Basic Black, Hot, Nude;* Joan Collins *Spectacular;* Salvador Dali *Parfum;* Daniel Fasson *Pour Femme;* Fendi *Asja;* Romeo Gigli; Kenize *Panourge;* Krizia *Uomo;* Lapidus *Pour Homme;* Lauren *Safari;* Léonard *Balahé;* Bob Mackie *Parfum;* Maxim's *Parfum and Pour Homme;* Moschino; de la Renta *Parfum;* Van Cleef and Arpels *First.* 22 items. Est. $175.00-$225.00.

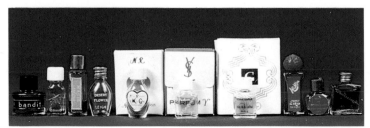

Lot #8. Lot of 10 miniature bottles, various heights from 1" to 1.7" [2.5 to 4.3 cm]: Ciro *Acclaim,* Desprez *Nuit de Versailles,* Lancôme *Magie,* Leigh *Desert Flower,* Lenthéric *Tweed,* Piguet *Bandit,* Rosenstein *Odalisque* and *Mlle. Ghe* in box, Saint Laurent *Y* in box, Guerlain *Chamade* in box. 10 items. Est. $100.00-$125.00.

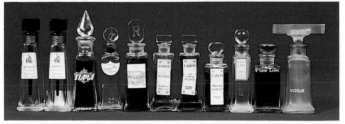

Lot #9. Glass testers with daubers: Lanvin *Prétexte* and *Rumeur* both with black stoppers, bottles marked Publicité; Corday *Toujours Moi;* Ciro *Camelia du Maroc;* Caron *Bellodgia, Le Tabac Blond* [label torn], *French Cancan;* Mary Chess *White Lilac;* Raphael *Plaisir* [label stain]; Vogue tester; Alexa *Tiara* [not a tester]. Eleven items. Est. $110.00-$165.00.

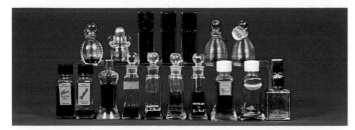

Lot #10. Miniatures & testers: Hattie Carnegie *Pink* [2], *Blue*; Yardley *Bond Street, April Violets*; Matchabelli *Abano, Stradivari, Crown Jewel*; Evyan *Most Precious*; Dunhill replica minis *Gardenia* [3, two without label]; Rosenstein all glass tester *Tianne*; Monteil *Nostalgia*, glass topped testers *Nostalgia, Rigolade, Gigolo*. 17 items. Est. $85.00-$170.00.

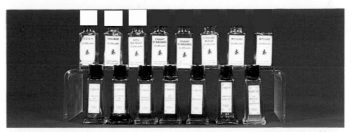

Lot #11. Guerlain 8 glass testers & black caps 2.4" [6.2 cm]: *Chant d'Arômes* [2], *Vol de Nuit, Shalimar, Mitsouko* [2], *L'Heure Bleue, Jicky* [label torn]; Caron 7 clear glass testers & gold caps 2.5" [6.3 cm]: *French Cancan, Fleurs de Rocaille, Nuit de Noël, Muguet de Bonheur, Pois de Senteur, Le Tabac Blond, Bellodgia*. 15 items. Est. $150.00-$250.00.

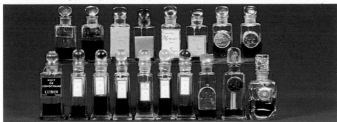

Lot #12. Lot of glass testers with glass tops: Ciro *New Horizons* [2], *Reflexions, Surrender* [2], *Danger*; Evyan *Enchanting Menace* [2], *Most Precious, Golden Shadows, Gay Diversion* [2]; Patou *Moment Supreme*; Rigaud *Un Air Embaumé*; Dana *20 Carats, Emir*; Lubin *Nuit de Lonchamps*; Ybry *Desir du Coeur*. 18 items. Est. $100.00-$200.00.

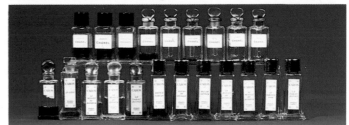

Lot #13. Caron 7 glass testers with gold caps: *Le Muguet* [2], *Fleurs de Rocaille, Pois de Senteur, French Cancan, Le Tabac Blond, Le Narcisse Noir*; 5 glass testers with glass tops: *Le Tabac Blond, Le Muguet* [2], one with torn label, *En Avion*; Chanel 6 glass testers with glass tops: *Jasmin* [2], *No. 5, No. 22, Gardenia, Russian Leather*; 3 glass testers with black caps: *Jasmin* [2]; *Russian Leather*. 21 items. Est. $105.00-$210.00.

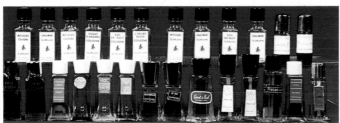

Lot #14. Lot of glass testers with screw-on caps: Guerlain *Vol de Nuit* [2], *Shalimar* [3], *Mitsouko* [3], *Chant d'Arômes, L'Heure Bleue*; Balenciaga *Le Dix, Quadrille*; Weil *Secret of Venus* [2]; Ricci *L'Air du Temps, Fille d'Eve*; Coty *L'Emeraude, L'Origan, L'Aimant*; Worth *Je Reviens, Oeillet*; Revillon *Carnet de Bal*; Piguet *Fracas*; Carven *Ma Griffe, Robe d'un Soir*; Vigny *Le Golliwogg*. 26 items. Est. $130.00-$260.00.

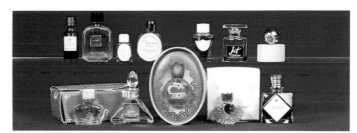

Lot #15. Ricci *L'Air du Temps* in box; Matchabelli *Golden Autumn* in box; Rubenstein *Apple Blossom* in windowed box; Dior *Miss Dior, Diorissimo*; La Prairie *One Perfect Rose*; Corday *Possession* and *Jet* with glass stopper; Molyneux *Rue Royale*; Arden *Night and Day* [glass stopper]; D'Orsay *Trophée*; Heim *Ariane*. 12 items. Est. $300.00-$400.00.

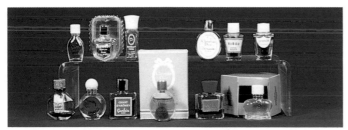

Lot #16. Lot of 12 minis: d'Albret *Ecusson* in plastic box; Corday *Jasmin*; Lily Daché *Dachelle*; Christian Dior *Diorissimo*, and *Miss Dior*, name in black enamel, in its box; d'Orsay *Le Dandy*; Guerlain *Chant d'Arômes*; Gould *#25*, Leigh *Heart Beat*; Matchabelli *Prophesy*, in its box; Odéon *Ribou*; Helena Rubenstein *Country*. 12 items. Est. $150.00-$250.00.

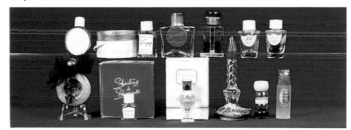

Lot #17. Lot of 12 minis: H. Carnegie *Parfum à Gogo* in hatbox; Corday *Jet, Lilas*; Goya *Heather*; Dior *Diorling* and *Miss Dior* in box; Schiaparelli *Sleeping* and *Shocking* in box; Dana *Bon Voyage*; Harriet Hubbard Ayer *Pink Clover*, Rochas *Femme*; Arden *Blue Grass*. 12 items. Est. $300.00-$400.00.

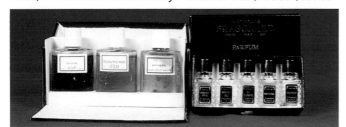

Lot #18. Fragonard *Natouna, Rendez-Vous, Murmure, Oui Madame, Moment Volé* clear glass bottles with black caps and labels, 1.5" [3.8 cm], in their black box; Violet *Chypre, Ecoutez-Moi, Apogée* clear glass bottles with white caps, 2.4" [6 cm], two with perfume, one with stained label, in their drop-front box [stains inside] also with label. Two boxed sets. Est. $75.00-$150.00.

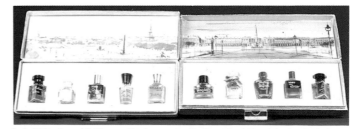

Lot #19. Les Meilleurs Parfums de Paris set of 5 minis in their box: Balmain *Jolie Madame*; Raphael *Réplique*; Dana *Tabu*; Capucci *Graffiti*; Pucci *Vivara*; Parfums de Paris set of 5 minis in their box: Piguet *Baghari*; Grès *Cabochard*; Schiaparelli *Shocking*; Dana *Tabu*; Balmain *Jolie Madame*. Two boxed sets. Est. $100.00-$175.00.

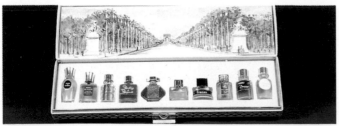

Lot #20. Les Parfums de Paris set of ten miniature glass bottles with gold or black caps: Corday *Fame;* De Rauch *Miss De Rauch;* Carven *Vert et Blanc;* Schiaparelli *Shocking;* Millot *Crêpe de Chine;* Revillon *Carnet de Bal;* Piguet *Fracas;* Le Galion *Sortilège;* Dana *Tabu;* Weil *Zibeline;* in a box marked #2. Est. $125.00-$175.00.

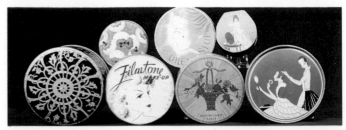

Lot #21. Lot of 7 fine powder boxes: Coty *Ambre Antique,* unused; Guerlain *Shalimar La Poudre C'est Moi,* unused; House of Hollywood *Filmtone* solid, some use; Richard Hudnut *Deauville* and *Three Flowers,* both unused; Houbigant *Le Parfum Idéal,* unused; Woodbury *Dream Stuff,* used. Seven items. Est. $140.00-$280.00.

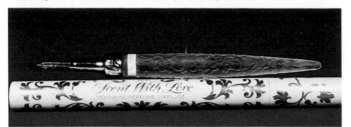

Lot #22. Avon *Moonwind* frosted glass bottle and gold cap in the shape of a fountain pen, 7" [17.8 cm], the bottle molded with an elaborate leaf design, full, label around bottle, in its cylindrical box marked "Scent with Love." Est. $40.00-$60.00.

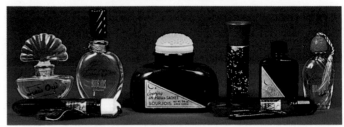

Lot #23. Bourjois *Mais Oui,* 2.4" [6 cm], *Courage* [2 diff.], 3.1" [8 cm] and 2.4" [6 cm], *Soir de Paris* mini/black cap, 2" [5.3 cm]; *Evening in Paris* tasseled purse vials [one with black cap, one with white cap], 3.2" [8.2 cm]; *E. I. P.* blue glass sachet with frosted top, and metal encased purse bottle with gold stars, label on bottom. 8 items. Est. $100.00-$175.00.

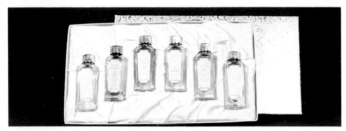

Lot #24. Mary Chess set of 6 toilet water miniatures: *Carnation, White Lilac, Yram, Gardenia, Tapestry, Strategy,* each glass bottle 2.4" [6.1 cm], gold caps, in a satin-lined gold foil presentation box. Est. $120.00-$180.00.

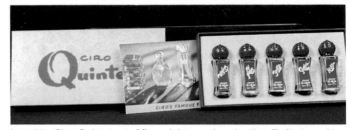

Lot #25. Ciro *Quintet* set of five miniature glass bottles *Reflexions, New Horizons, Danger, Surrender, Acclaim,* 1.8" [4.5 cm], each with rose-form red plastic caps, red labels, in a box with a colorful promotional pamphlet advertising the standard bottles. Est. $100.00-$150.00.

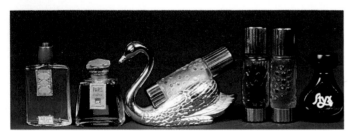

Lot #26. Coty various miniatures: *Styx* black glass bottle and cap, *Emeraude* with green cap, *Paris* with frosted glass stopper, *L'Aimant* [2] and *Emeraude* frosted glass bottles of lipstick shape with brass caps, one of which is mounted in a plastic swan, various heights from 1.7" to 2.5" [4.3 cm to 6.4 cm]. Six items. Est. $60.00-$120.00.

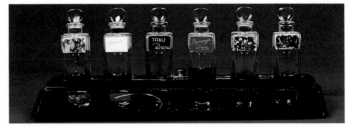

Lot #27. Dana set of 6 glass tester bottles with glass stoppers and daubers: *Emir, Ambush, Tabu, Bon Voyage, Platine, 20 Carats,* mounted in a black plastic stand marked Dana. Est. $125.00-$200.00.

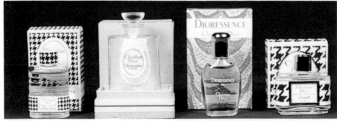

Lot #28. Christian Dior lot of four boxed miniatures: *Miss Dior,* glass bottle with white cap, 1.9" [4.8 cm]; *Dioressence,* glass bottle with gold cap, 2.4" [6 cm]; *Diorella,* glass bottle with silver cap, 1.7" [4.3 cm]; all with their perfume; *Diorissimo* clear glass bottle and glass stopper, 2.4" [6 cm]. Four items. Est. $150.00-$300.00.

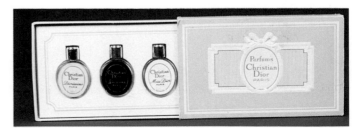

Lot #29. Christian Dior *Diorissimo, Diorama, Miss Dior* set of three glass miniature bottles with brass caps, each 1.6" [4 cm], each bottle the *galet* or 'cobblestone' shape and each molded France on back, all in their gray and white box. Est. $250.00-$350.00.

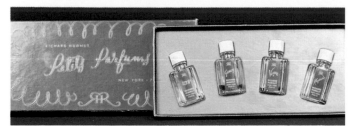

Lot #30. Richard Hudnut *Petits Parfums: Gemey, RSVP, Rhapsody, Vogue* set of four glass bottles with white plastic caps, 1.7" [4.3 cm], each with a pink label, in their pink box and outer cover. Est. $100.00-$150.00.

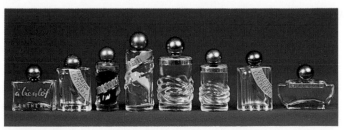

Lot #31. Lenthéric lot of eight: *Repartée* [two sizes], *Violette, Carnation, Confetti* [two sizes], *A Bientôt, Shanghai,* all replica glass miniatures with gold ball-shaped caps, sizes from 1.3" to 2.2" [3.3 to 5.6 cm], all but one empty. Eight items. Est. $80.00-$160.00.

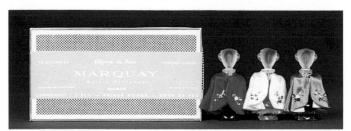

Lot #32. Marquay *L'Elu* ['The Chosen'], *Prince Douka, Coup de Feu* ['Gunshot'] clear glass rectangular bottles and frosted glass stoppers, 2.8" [7.1 cm], the stoppers molded in a highly stylized depiction of a head [unlike the usual realistic stoppers], red, white and blue capes, full and sealed, gold labels around neck, in their box.   Est. $250.00-$350.00.

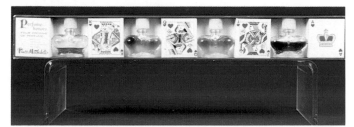

Lot #33. Matchabelli "Perfume Honors - Four Crowns of Perfume" *Windsong, Stradivari, Added Attraction, Beloved* clear glass miniature bottles with white gold-flecked caps, each 1.3" [3.4 cm], in a long box with the king, queen, jack, and ace of hearts. Est. $150.00-$250.00.

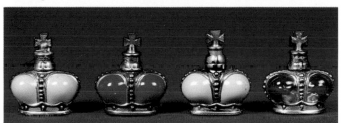

Lot #34. Matchabelli *Added Attraction* [red], *Beloved* [blue], *Stradivari* [clear], *Windsong* [green] clear glass crown bottles and cross stoppers, each 1.9" [4.7 cm], enameled colors, empty, labels on bottom [label for blue one lacking]. Four items. Est. $275.00-$400.00.

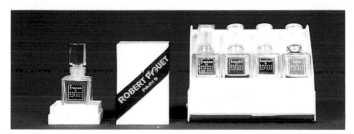

Lot #35. Robert Piguet *Futur, Baghari, Fracas, Bandit,* set of four glass bottles with glass stoppers, each 2.3" [5.8 cm], black labels, some perfume in an interesting ensemble presentation [minor stains]; *Fracas,* same size, empty, in its separate box; probably all first sizes. Five bottles. Est. $125.00-$150.00.

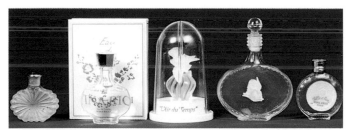

Lot #36. Nina Ricci *L'Air du Temps* clear glass bottle and stopper of oval shape with long neck and ball stopper, 3.3" [8.4 cm], empty, label, bottom signed Lalique; *L'Air du Temps* frosted glass bottle and brass cap, 1.6" [4 cm], sunburst shape, and glass bottle with plastic bird stopper, 1.8" [4.6 cm], in its plastic dome; *Fille d'Eve* glass bottle with gold cap, 2" [5 cm], label, empty; *Eau de Fleurs* glass bottle with gold cap, 2.2" [5.5 cm], full, in its box. Five items. Est. $150.00-$225.00.

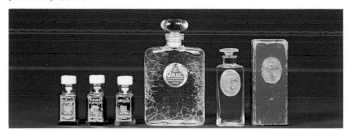

Lot #37. Roger & Gallet *Le Jade, Santalia, Fleurs d'Amour* clear glass bottles with white tester caps marked RG, 1.7" [4.3 cm] each, gold labels, full; *Fleurs d'Amour* glass bottle and stopper, 2.8" [7 cm], gold label with an angel, in its box [worn]; *Le Jade* crackle glass bottle and stopper, 3.7" [9.5 cm], empty, label with birds. Five items. Est. $200.00-$275.00.

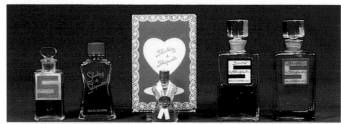

Lot #38. Schiaparelli *Shocking* glass mini with brass cap, 1.6" [4 cm], clean tape measure label, unused, in its pink box; *Soucis* and *Shocking* glass bottles and cube stoppers, 3" [7.8 cm], unopened, [pink label stained]; *Shocking* clear glass bottle and stopper, 2.4" [6 cm], pink cap, names in pink enamel; *Succès Fou* glass tester with dauber, 2.3" [5.8 cm]. Five items. Est. $175.00-$250.00.

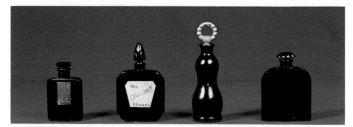

Lot #39. Char'net *May Blossoms* black glass bottle and stopper, 2.9" [7.4 cm], empty, silver label; d'Orsay *Le Dandy* black glass bottle and stopper, 2.5" [6.4 cm], label lacking, empty; Lily *Bermuda* black glass bottle and stopper with dauber, 2.2" [5.6 cm], gold label, empty; Rosenfeld glass bottle enameled black and stopper enameled gold, label on bottom, empty. Four items. Est. $200.00-$250.00.

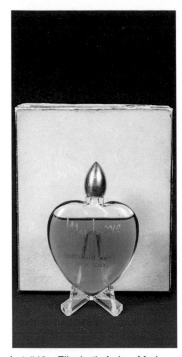

Lot #40. Elizabeth Arden *My Love* rare and unusual clear glass bottle with brass cap, 2.7" [6.9 cm], the bottle of heart shape, names in gold enamel on front, with perfume, in its cream and gold box. Est. $150.00-$250.00.

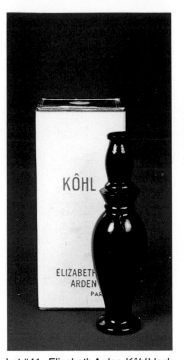

Lot #41. Elizabeth Arden *Kôhl* black glass bottle and stopper, 2.8" [7.2 cm], the bottle an interesting urn shape, for dispensing eye make-up, bottom molded Arden France, in a gold and cream box. Est. $100.00-$150.00.

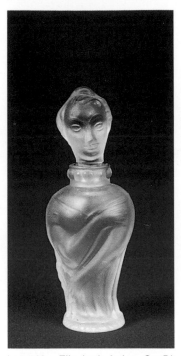

Lot #42. Elizabeth Arden *On Dit* frosted glass bottle in the form of a woman, the stopper molded as the head, 2.9" [7.4 cm], label [worn, faint] on bottom, empty, probably a first size. Est. $200.00-$250.00.

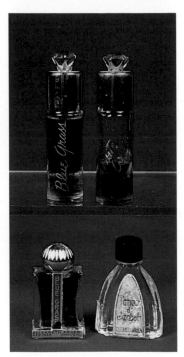

Lot #43. Elizabeth Arden *Blue Grass* and *White Orchid*, clear glass bottles with brass cap and colored stones, 2.8" [7 cm], names in gold; *L'Amour d'Elizabeth* with black cap, 1.8" [4.5 cm], empty [worn label]; *Blue Grass* glass replica mini with gold cap, 1.7" [4.2 cm]. Four miniatures. Est. $75.00-$100.00.

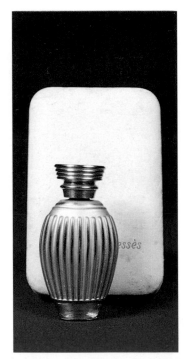

Lot #44. Jean Dessès *Celui* gold enameled glass bottle and gold metal cap, 2" [5.1 cm], the ribbed shape replica of the standard bottle, 1/8th oz. size, in its satin lined box. Est. $125.00-$175.00.

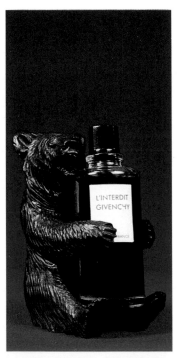

Lot #45. Givenchy *L'Interdit* ['The Forbidden'] clear glass bottle and black cap, 3.3" [8.4 cm], standard cylinder bottle, full, label, held in the arms of a bear made of composition. Est. $50.00-$100.00.

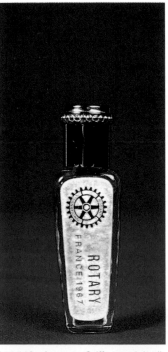

Lot #46. Jacques Griffe special edition clear glass miniature bottle and gold cap, 2.4" [6.2 cm], the bottle with rows of indented beads, full, label marked Rotary International France 1967. Est. $50.00-$100.00.

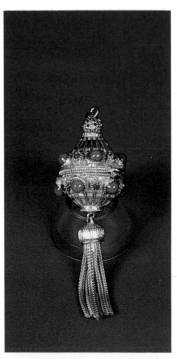

Lot #47. Costume jewelry perfume pendant, 3" [7.6 cm] to end of tassel, designed as a miniature pomander and mounted with red and green stones, loop at top for necklace, hinges open at middle, inside marked Florenz. Est. $50.00-$100.00.

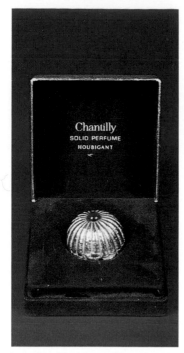

Lot #48. Houbigant *Chantilly* solid perfume gold metal container, 1.2" [3 cm], of ball shape with a ribbed design and topped with a red stone, unused, Houbigant molded inside, with tiny label on bottom, in its fitted box. Est. $50.00-$85.00.

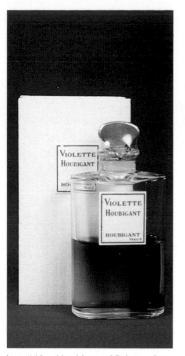

Lot #49. Houbigant *Violette* clear glass bottle and stopper, 2.7" [6.9 cm], of oval shape with gold enameled stopper, violet label, some perfume and sealed, in its box with identical label, polished bottom acid marked France. Est. $60.00-$85.00.

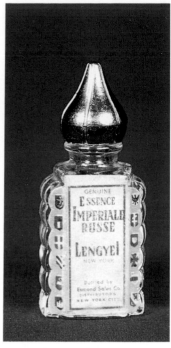

Lot #50. Lengyel *Essence Impériale Russe* glass bottle and metal cap, 2" [5.1 cm], the bottle made to resemble the architectural form of a Russian cathedral with onion dome, empty, colorful label on front. Est. $100.00-$125.00.

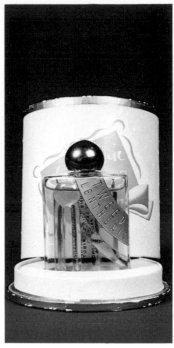

Lot #51. Lenthéric *Tweed* clear glass bottle and gold metal ball cap, 2" [5.1 cm], gold label on front, full, in its tiny original blue and violet box. Est. $60.00-$85.00.

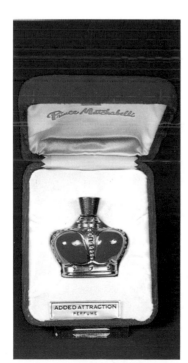

Lot #52. Matchabelli *Added Attraction*, glass bottle with gold screw-on cap, 1.6" (4 cm), the bottle enameled in red and gold, gold oval label on bottom, in its original presentation box of red velvet lined with white satin. Est. $200.00-$350.00.

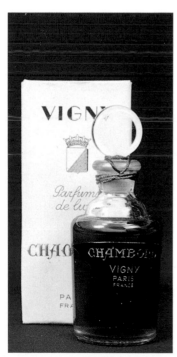

Lot #53. Vigny *Chambord* clear glass bottle and stopper, 2.9" [7.4 cm], apothecary shape, full and sealed, black label, in its original box; this perfume bears the name of a beautiful French castle, and box reads "Le roi festoie parfum de joie de pourpre et d'or..." ['The King regales with perfume of joy of purple and gold...']. Est. $75.00-$125.00.

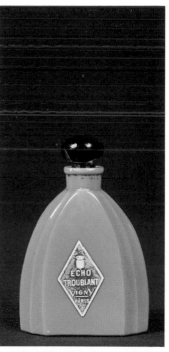

Lot #54. Vigny *Echo Troublant* green opaque glass bottle and clear green stopper, 2.2" [5.5 cm], empty, label also greenish and gold, empty, bottom molded France. Est. $200.00-$300.00.

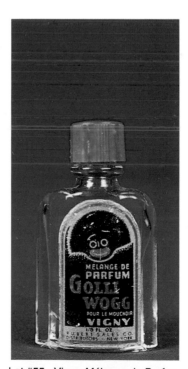

Lot #55. Vigny *Mélange de Parfum Le Golliwogg* pour le mouchoir ['...for the handkerchief'], rare glass miniature bottle and red cap, 2" [5.1 cm], Golliwogg on the front label, empty. Est. $100.00-$200.00.

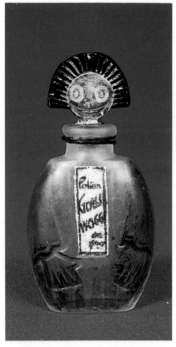

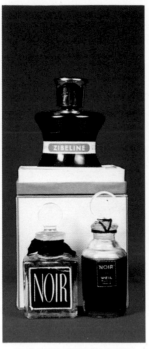

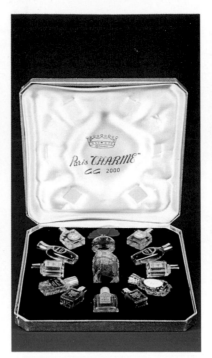

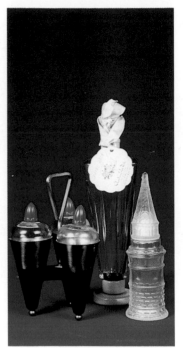

Lot #56. Vigny *Le Golliwogg* extremely rare and early frosted glass bottle and black glass stopper, 2.5" [6.4 cm], the bottle of flat oval shape molded as a standing Golliwogg with hands at side, stopper with paper label face and long dauber [top edge with small smoothed spot], label [worn] on front, traces of black patina. Cf. Lefkowith, p. 71, #55. Est. $300.00-$400.00.

Lot #57. Weil *Zibeline* ['Sable'] *Secret of Venus* clear glass bottle with brass cap, 2" [5.1 cm], spool shape, full, label, in its box; *Noir* ['Black'] two different clear glass bottles and stoppers, 2.1" [5.3 cm] and 2.3" [5.8 cm], full, black labels. Three items. Est. $75.00-$125.00.

Lot #58. *Paris Charme* set of 13 miniature bottles: Piguet *Bandit* [2], Marquay *Coup de Feu*, Vigny *Heure Intime*, Houbigant *Essence Rare*, Folies Bergere, Berdoes *Capri, Cordoba, Tonka, Ambre, Tabac, Joie, Smyr;* all arranged clockform in a gold hinged presentation case. Est. $100.00-$150.00.

Lot #59. Charles of the Ritz *Spring Rain* glass bottle shaped as an umbrella, wood cap and base, 8.4" [21.3 cm], label with ribbon, empty; *Morning, Noon, Nite* clear glass bottles, red caps in a metal tripod; Novaya Zarya *Kreml* ['New Dawn: Kremlin'] frosted glass bottle, white cap, and glass overcap shaped as a Kremlin tower, empty, gold label. Three items. Est. $50.00-$75.00.

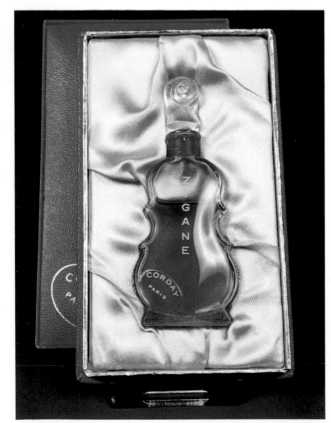

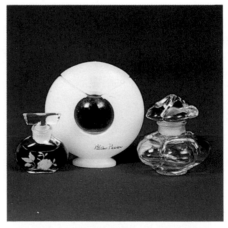

Lot #61. Paloma Picasso miniature glass bottle in white plastic casing, 2.2" [5.6 cm], *Flora Danica*, 1.3" [3.3 cm], Corday *Orchidée Bleue* clear glass bottle and stopper, 1.7" [4.3 cm], empty [no label]. Three items. Est. $75.00-$125.00.

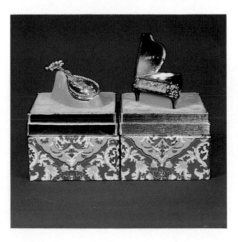

Lot #62. Avon *Brocade* Perfume Glacé gold metal Mandolin for solid perfume, 2.4" long [6.1 cm], unused, in its box; *Brocade* Perfume Glacé gold metal baby grand piano, 1" [2.5 cm], unused, in its fitted box. Two items. Est. $50.00-$80.00.

Lot #60. Corday *Zigane* 1/5 oz. clear glass bottle and ground glass stopper in the shape of a violin, 3" [7.6 cm], name in gold enamel, Corday written on the chin rest, with perfume, in its deep pink box with pink satin lining. Est. $125.00-$175.00.

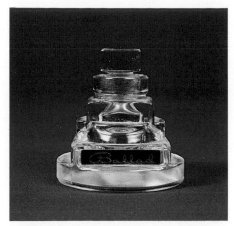

Lot #63. Avon *Ballad* clear glass bottle and stopper, 1.8" [4.5 cm], in the form of a pyramid created by stacked circles and squares, gold metallic labels front and back. Est. $75.00-$125.00.

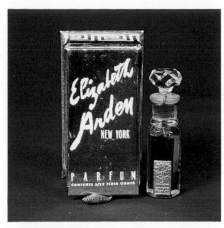

Lot #64. Elizabeth Arden *Cupid's Breath* clear glass bottle and stopper, 2.4" [6 cm], the bottle a hexagonal column, faceted stopper, gold label, full and sealed, in a beautiful little gold and white box with a Greek key design, with outer box. Est. $125.00-$175.00.

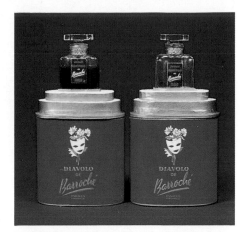

Lot #65. Barroché *Diavolo* pair of identical clear glass bottles and stoppers, 2.1" [5.3 cm], script B molded into stopper, bottom molded Barroché and France, one full and sealed, one empty, in their beautiful red boxes with mask and flowers. Two items. Est. $75.00-$125.00.

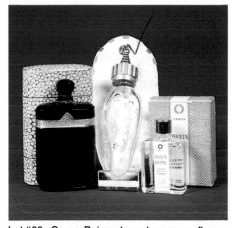

Lot #66. Caron *Poivre* clear glass purse flacon with gold metal cap, 3.5" [8.9 cm], the bottle with indented dots, empty, in its white leather pouch; *Nuit de Noël* black glass bottle and stopper, 2.7" [6.9 cm], prob. a first size, label, empty, in its faux shagreen box; *Pour Un Homme* glass bottle and metal cap, 1.8" [4.6 cm], full, label, in its box. Three items. Est. $75.00-$100.00.

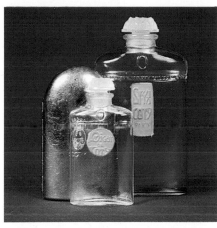

Lot #67. Coty *Styx* clear glass bottle and stopper of flask shape, 3.5" [8.9 cm], stopper molded with flowers, gold label, empty, bottom signed Coty; *L'Origan* clear glass bottle and stopper of identical design, 2.2" [5.6 cm], empty, gold label, in its metal carrying case with Coty logo. Two items. Est. $100.00-$150.00.

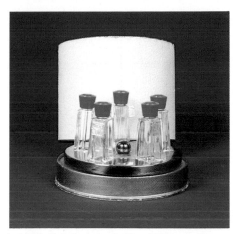

Lot #68. Coty tester set of five *L'Aimant, Chypre, Paris, Emeraude, Muguet*: clear glass bottles with red caps, 2.5" (6.4 cm), empty, with glass daubers, in a carousel of brass in a round box. Est. $150.00-$225.00.

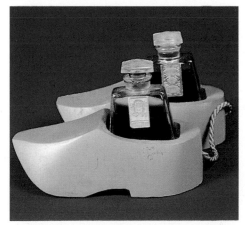

Lot #69. Coty *Emeraude* and *L'Aimant* pair of clear glass bottles with frosted glass stoppers, 1.8" [4.5 cm] each sitting in a wooden shoe tied together by a cord, stoppers with fishscale motif, with labels, full and sealed. Est. $125.00-$175.00.

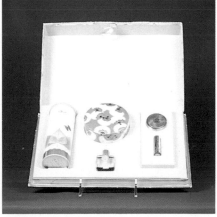

Lot #70. Coty *L'Origan* gift set consisting of talc, unopened powder decorated with puffs, perfume miniature with brass cap, 1.8" [4.5 cm], lipstick *Sub-Deb* in brass case, small brass compact, all in a box decorated with leaves on a silver background. Est. $100.00-$125.00.

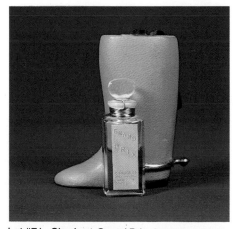

Lot #71. Charbert *Grand Prix* clear glass tester bottle and stopper with dauber, 2.4" [6 cm], near full and sealed, an unusual presentation in a leather boot, also stamped on sole Charbert *Grand Prix*. Est. $75.00-$100.00.

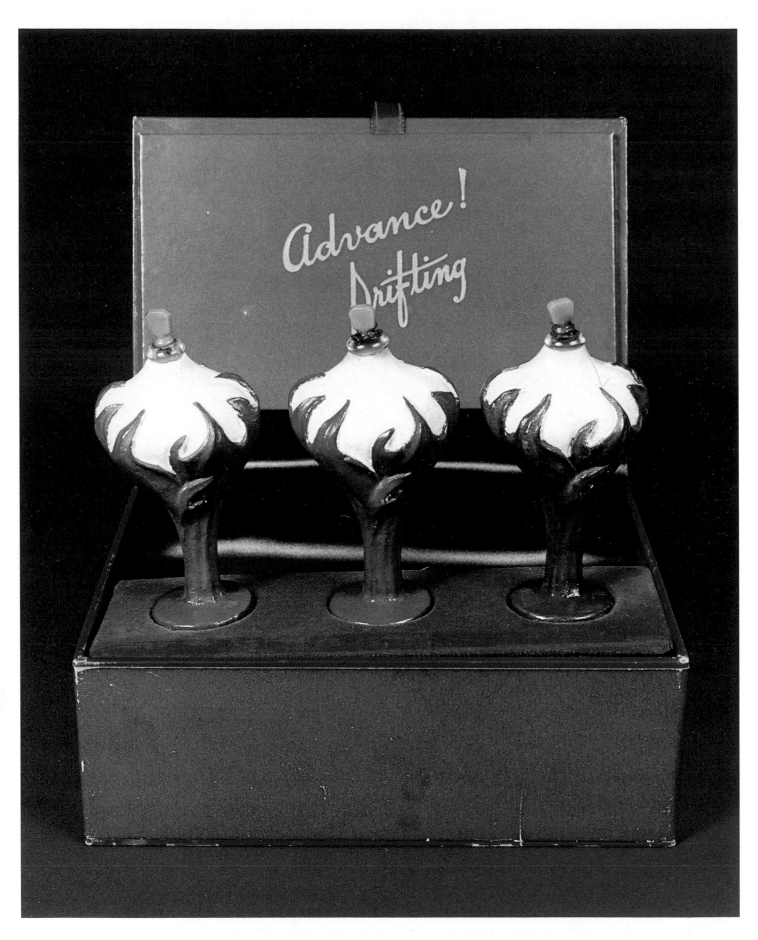

Lot #72. Lily Daché *Drifting* unusual and very rare set of three small bottles made of glass and mounted in a composition form resembling a woman's bosom, green plastic stoppers, mounted as a trio in a beautiful green and pink box with green satin interior. Cf. Lefkowith, p. 18, #2. Est. $1200.00-$1500.00.

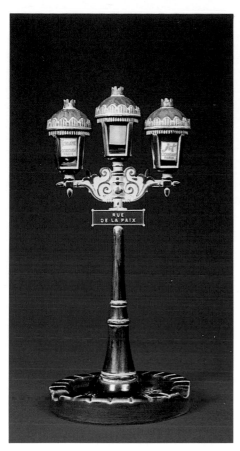

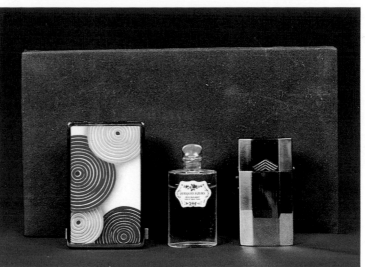

Lot #74. Houbigant *Quelques Fleurs* ['Some Flowers'] clear glass bottle and stopper, 2.4" [6.1 cm], full and sealed, stopper with gold enamel, label, in a brass carrying case; stunning compact with two powders and tiny lipstick, all unused, compact with a beautiful abstract design in red, green, and white; in a dark blue flocked box with white satin lining. Est. $250.00-$350.00.

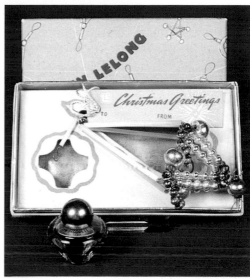

Lot #73. Corday *Ardente Nuit, Jet, Tsigane* set of three glass bottles with gold caps, each 1.4" [3.6 cm], in their original lamppost holder commemorating the Rue de la Paix with ceramic ashtray base marked Corday Paris on bottom. Est. $250.00-$350.00.

Lot #75. Richard Hudnut *Le Début Noir* black glass bottle and stopper, 1.4" [3.5 cm], of flat octagonal shape, stopper with gilding, tiny gold label [letters faint], full and sealed. Est. $300.00-$400.00.

Lot #76. Lucien Lelong *Indiscrete* [sic] rare and unusual clear glass miniature bottle with brass ball cap, 1.1" [2.8 cm], the flower pot-shaped bottle with indented portions on four sides, gold label on shoulder, in a beaded ornament holder [marked Czechoslovakia] to be hung on the Christmas tree, gift tag included, in its box. Est. $125.00-$175.00.

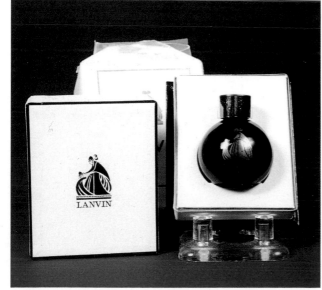

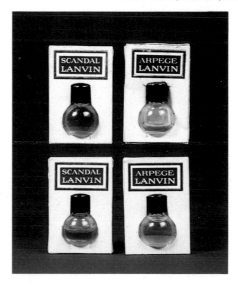

Lot #78. Lanvin *Arpège* [2] and *Scandal* [2] miniature glass bottles with black caps, 1" [2.5 cm], the bottle a replica shape of the classic boule, each in a small cardboard holder printed on back: *Voici Madame l'occasion d'apprécier l'un des délicieux parfums créés pour vous par Lanvin* ['Here, Madame, is the chance to sample one of the delicious perfumes created for you by Lanvin']. Four items. Est. $200.00-$300.00.

Lot #77. Lanvin *Arpège* deluxe black glass miniature boule with brass cap, 1.2" [3 cm], name and logo enameled in gold in front, in its tiny box and outer paper marked *Offert Gratieusement* ['Free Gift']. Est. $800.00-$1000.00.

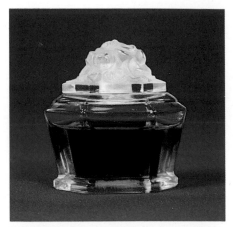

Lot #79. Maudy *Jasmin* clear glass bottle, inner stopper, and frosted glass overcap, 2.2" [5.6 cm], the overcapr molded as a bouquet of flowers, with perfume, label on bottom, probably a first size. Est. $125.00-$200.00.

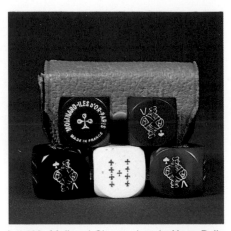

Lot #80. Molinard *Chypre, Jasmin, Xmas Bells, Fleurettes, Iles d'Or* set of five bakelite dice for solid perfume, each .7" [1.8 cm], the dice white, blue, black, deep red, and green; and with card denominations on various sides [Queen of hearts, ten, etc.], in their small leather pouch also marked Molinard. Est. $125.00-$175.00.

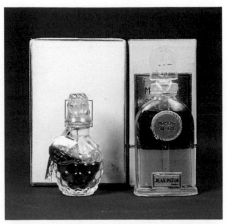

Lot #81. Jean Patou *Moment Suprême* clear glass bottle and stopper, 2.2" [5.5 cm], both bottle and stopper molded with round cabochons, full and sealed, gold label around neck, in its box; clear glass bottle and stopper with long dauber, 3.2" [8.1 cm], full and sealed, JP logo on stopper, gold labels, in its box. Two items. Est. $175.00-$250.00.

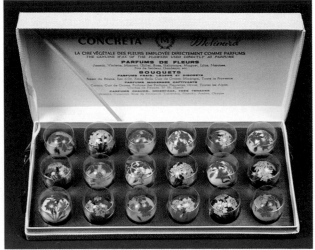

Lot #82. Molinard *Oeillet* ['Carnation'] *Concréta* set of 18 mulitcolor bakelite containers of ball shape on black base, each colorfully hand-painted with three carnations, labels on bottom, each in a celluloid container in their box and outer cover. Est. $275.00-$375.00.

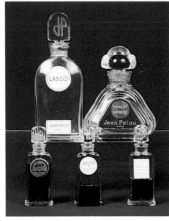

Lot #83. Jean Patou *Joy, Lasso, Joy Eau* glass testers + daubers, each 2.8" [7.1 cm], labels; *Lasso* similar shape larger glass bottle, 4.7" [12 cm]; *Moment Suprême* clear glass bottle and stopper, 3.5" [9 cm], empty, label on front. 5 items. Est. $125.00-$175.00.

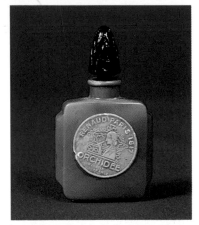

Lot #84. Renaud *Orchidée* violet opaque glass bottle with black glass stopper, 2.1" [5.3 cm], empty, beautiful gold label on front. Est. $150.00-$250.00.

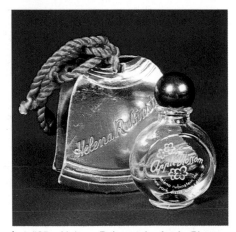

Lot #85. Helena Rubenstein *Apple Blossom* clear glass miniature perfume bottle with gold metal ball cap, 1.6" [4 cm], names in enamel on front, in an unusual box shaped as a bell in which the perfume bottle is upside down and the gold cap appears as the bell's clapper. Est. $125.00-$200.00.

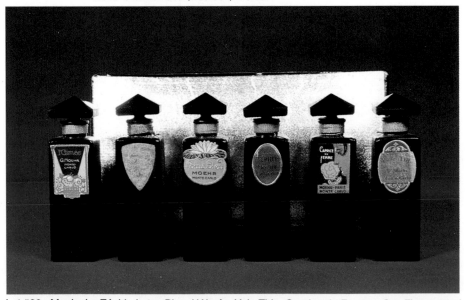

Lot #86. Moehr *Le Zéphir, Lotus Bleu, L'Aimée, Yule Tide, Caprice de Femme, Ses Fleurs* set of six black glass bottles and stoppers, each 3.1" [8 cm], stoppers of pyramid shape, all full and sealed, each with a beautiful label, in a beautiful gold foil box marked "Purveyors to the King of England and the Prince of Monaco." Est. $450.00-$550.00.

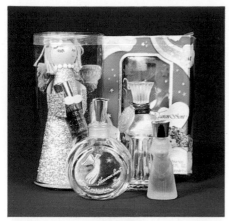

Lot #87. Helena Rubenstein *Heaven Sent* two different clear glass bottles and stoppers, 3.3" [8.4 cm] & 3.7" [9.4 cm], empty; cylinder bottle with gold cap, 2.5" [6.4 cm], held by a paper angel; frosted glass bottle in the shape of an angel, 2.6" [6.6 cm], full, label on bottom, in its original box. Four items. Est. $125.00-$175.00.

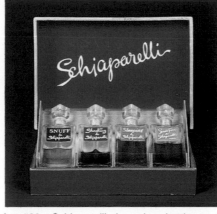

Lot #88. Schiaparelli clear glass bottles and glass stoppers: *Snuff, Shocking, Sleeping, Succès Fou*, each 2.4" [6.1 cm], bottles of rectangular form with cube stoppers having long daubers, labels in the signature color of each fragrance [brown, pink, blue, green], full and sealed, in their pink box. Est. $175.00-$225.00.

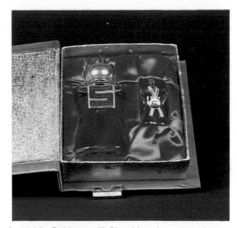

Lot #89. Schiaparelli *Shocking* clear glass bottle with gold ball cap, 4" [10.2 cm], "S" label on front, full; miniature dress form glass bottle with brass cap, 2" [5.1 cm], label around neck, full, both bottles in a pink satin lined book-form box marked "Gift from Paris Deluxe Edition." Est. $200.00-$300.00.

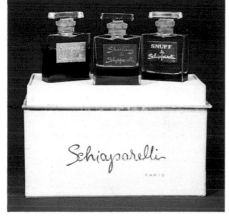

Lot #90. Schlaparelli *Snuff, Sleeping, Shocking* set of three small rectangular bottles, each 1.9" [4.8 cm], with their red, brown, and blue labels, partial perfume but sealed, in a box marked Schiaparelli [stains to box top]. Est. $100.00-$125.00.

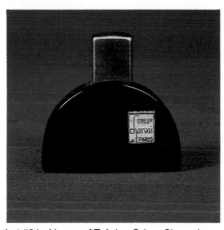

Lot #91. House of Tré-Jur *Odeur Charvai* rare black glass bottle, black glass inner stopper, and metal overcap, 1.6" [4 cm], tiny label on the side, identifying label also on bottom, empty. Est. $150.00-$250.00.

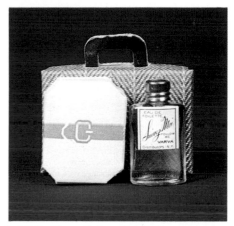

Lot #92. Varva *Suivez Moi* ['Follow Me'] clear glass miniature with brass cap, 1.5" [3.8 cm], miniature face powder, in a small cardboard suitcase. Est. $75.00-$100.00.

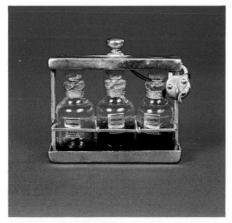

Lot #93. Weil *Bamboo, Zibeline, Cassandra* three clear glass bottles and stoppers with molded W, 2.3" [5.8 cm], all sealed, gold labels, in a tiny brass holder with lock and key. Est. $125.00-$200.00.

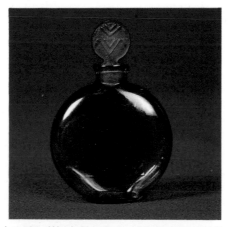

Lot #94. Worth *Vers le Jour* ['Toward the Day'] amber glass bottle and stopper, 2" [5.2 cm], the bottle of clear amber with the word Worth molded in front, the stopper frosted with a design of rows of chevrons, empty, bottom marked Paris France. Est. $150.00-$250.00.

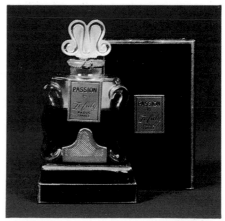

Lot #95. Zofaly *Passion* clear glass bottle and frosted glass stopper, 2.4" [6.1 cm], designed with swirled lines, with perfume and sealed, gold label, in a black box also with gold label; probably a first size. Est. $100.00-$150.00.

FACTICE - DISPLAY BOTTLES
MEMORABILIA -
PERFUME LAMPS

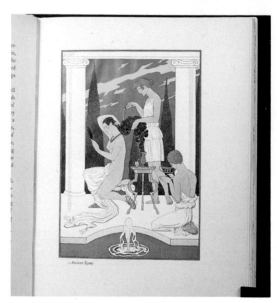

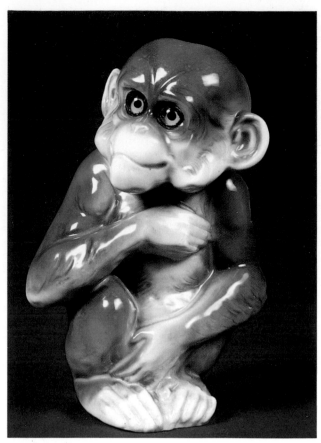

Lot #96. *The Romance of Perfume* by Richard Le Gallienne, beautifully illustrated with drawings by George Barbier, including an inner booklet "At 20 Rue de la Paix" about the Richard Hudnut Paris store; totally pristine condition. Est. $175.00-$225.00.

Lot #97. Large porcelain perfume lamp in the shape of a monkey, 7.5" [19 cm], the monkey realistically painted in brown and cream having a distinctly human-like face, yellow glass eyes, well for perfume in top of head, wired for electricity, "crown over N" mark inside, probably of German manufacture. Est. $300.00-$400.00.

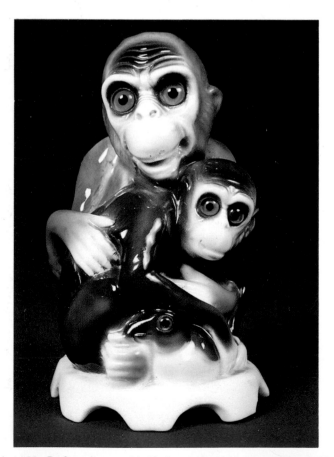

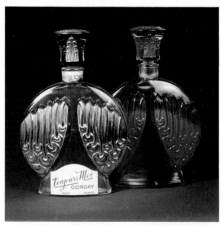

Lot #99. Corday *Toujours Moi* pair of clear glass bottles and stoppers, 8.7" [22 cm], with molded botanical decoration on bottles and stoppers, one with the design enameled in gold, label at base, empty; the other bottle with the design in red, no label, empty, both with bottom signed Corday. Two items. Est. $350.00-$450.00.

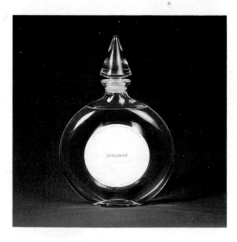

Lot #100. Guerlain *Shalimar* clear glass bottle and stopper, 9.4" [24 cm], round shape with indented center for label, cone stopper, full, label on front, marked dummy on back of label. Est. $100.00-$175.00.

Lot #98. Perfume lamp molded in the shape of a brown monkey holding a smaller gray monkey who in turn is holding a cockatoo, 5.3" [13.5 cm], all three animals with glass eyes, well in back for perfume, inside molded Aroma 29470, electrical fixture lacking. Est. $275.00-$375.00.

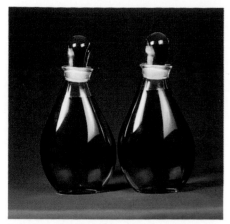

Lot #101. Halston pair of identical clear glass factice bottles, 10.7" [27.2 cm], designed by Elsa Peretti in the famous 'bean' shape, plastic tipped stoppers, circa 1960's. Two items. Est. $300.00-$400.00.

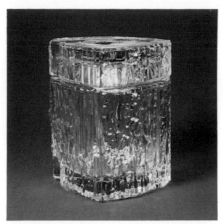

Lot #102. Houbigant *Essence Rare* clear glass bottle and stopper, 6.3" [16 cm], the entire bottle with basically three sides and resembling fractured ice, empty, silver label on top, bottom signed Houbigant. Est. $200.00-$300.00.

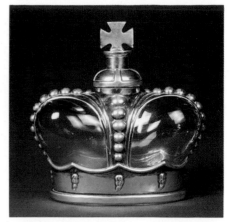

Lot #103. Matchabelli huge size clear glass bottle and glass stopper, 8" [20.3 cm], heavily enameled in gold and with black patina applied in the recesses, empty, bottom signed Prince Matchabelli. Est. $500.00-$600.00.

CROWN TOP

PORCELAIN

19TH CENTURY

DEVILBISS

ART GLASS

MURANO

DAUM

BACCARAT

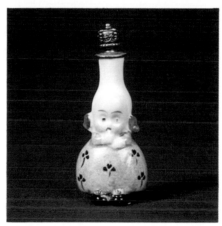

Lot #104. Ceramic bottle and metal crown stopper, 3" [7.6 cm], molded as a baby girl with thumb at mouth, painted brightly in green, yellow, pink and black, bottom marked Bavaria. Est. $100.00-$150.00.

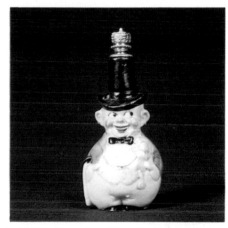

Lot #105. Ceramic bottle and metal crown stopper in the form of a fat little gentleman, 3.3" [8.4 cm], the man dressed in a suit with cane, lapel flower, and watch fob, the whole brightly painted, mold numbers 5783, bottom marked Germany in red. Est. $100.00-$150.00.

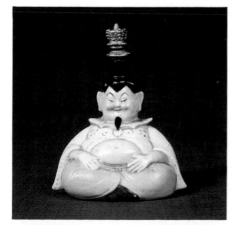

Lot #106. Ceramic bottle and metal crown stopper in the shape of a fat oriental potentate, 3" [7.5 cm], beautifully and realistically painted in blue, green, white, black, and flesh tones, back with mold #1709, of German manufacture. Est. $125.00-$175.00.

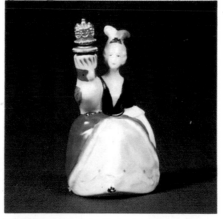

Lot #107. Ceramic bottle and metal crown stopper in the shape of a seated lady holding a huge parrot 3" [7.5 cm], beautifully and realistically painted in blue, red, white, black, and yellow, bottom stamped Germany in red enamel. Est. $100.00-$150.00.

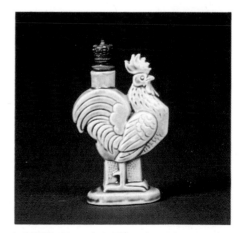

Lot #108. Ceramic bottle and metal crown stopper in the shape of a standing rooster, 2.8" [7 cm], light brown glaze, unsigned but of German manufacture. Est. $75.00-$125.00.

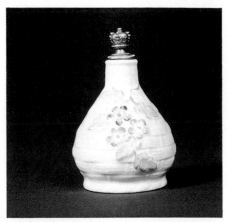

Lot #109. Crown Devon porcelain perfume bottle with metal crown stopper, 3.4" [8.6 cm], of beehive shape molded with a basket weave design and decorated with flowers, bottom with impressed number A-283, and signed Crown Devon England. Est. $100.00-$150.00.

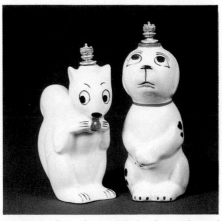

Lot #110. Pair of porcelain bottles and metal crown stoppers in the shape of a standing dog, 4.8" [12.2 cm], and a squirrel, 4.4" [11.2 cm], both decorated in red, black, and pink, bottom marked Garnier France, apparently produced originally for liquor. Two items. Est. $150.00-$250.00.

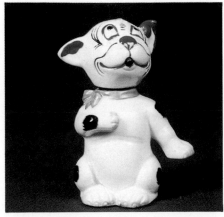

Lot #111. Porcelain two-piece atomizer in the shape of an adorable puppy with a fly on his head, 3.9" [10 cm], atomizer bulb fits into dogs head in the back, bottom molded Germany 6340. Est. $100.00-$125.00.

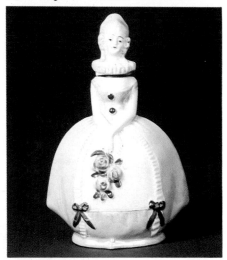

Lot #112. Porcelain figural perfume bottle, 6.2" [15.7 cm], in the form of a nineteenth century woman in a green and white ball gown holding a bouquet of roses, stopper at neckline with long glass dauber, mold #5924 on back, bottom marked Germany. Est. $125.00-$175.00.

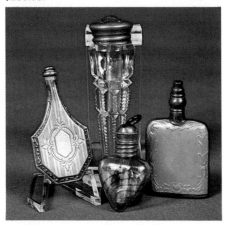

Lot #113. Clear cut crystal purse bottle with brass metal cap, 2.7" [6.9 cm]; tiny clear glass heart-shaped bottle with blue swirls 1.4" [3.7 cm], metal cap with loop, glass inner stopper [chip to neck]; silver metal purse bottle, 1.9" [4.8 cm]; pink enamel on brass purse bottle, 2" [5.1 cm]. Four items. Est. $50.00-$100.00.

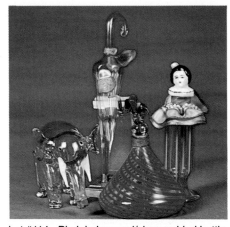

Lot #114. Bimini glass red/clear swirled bottle, 3.1" [8 cm], elephant stopper with dauber, paper label Germany; clear glass elephant, white tusks, 2.2" [5.5 cm], cork stopper; clear and swirled glass bottle with porcelain clown stopper, 3.7" [9.4 cm]; *Rose Perfume* glass umbrella, 4.8" [12.2 cm] cork stopper, unopened, labeled Germany. Four items. Est. $150.00-$250.00.

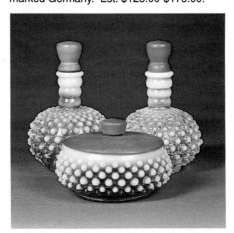

Lot #115. Wrisley *Gardenia* pair of opalescent glass cologne bottles with wood tops and wood-covered powder box, 6" tall [15.2 cm], partial label on bottom of one bottle, each in the hobnail pattern made by the Fenton Co. Set of three items. Est. $100.00-$150.00.

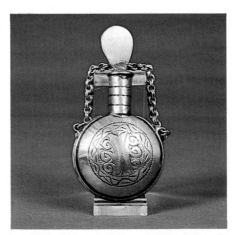

Lot #116. Unusual silver metal hand-wrought bottle, 3.5" [8.9 cm], screw-on stopper with dauber, metal chain attached on two sides of bottle, decorative motifs hammered onto both sides, probably of Middle Eastern or North African manufacture. Est. $100.00-$150.00.

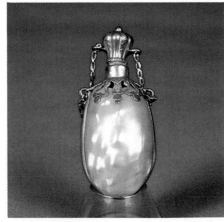

Lot #117. Mother of pearl perfume bottle, 2.5" [6.4 cm], egg-shaped and mounted with gold metal cork-tipped stopper and chains so as to be wearable, country of origin unidentified. Est. $100.00-$175.00.

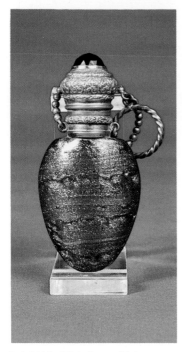

Lot #118. Victorian goldstone perfume bottle with silver colored metal mount, 3" [7.6 cm], oval shape with brilliant variations of gold and flecks of black, hinged lid with glass inner stopper and dauber, faceted violet stone mounted in the lid, chain attached with loop. Est. $200.00-$275.00.

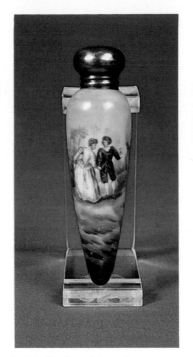

Lot #119. Porcelain perfume purse bottle, 3" [7.6 cm], the front painted with a lady and a gentleman on a light brown background, sterling silver top with English hallmarks for Birmingham, 1904, probably originally sold at the St. Louis World's Fair. Est. $150.00 $200.00.

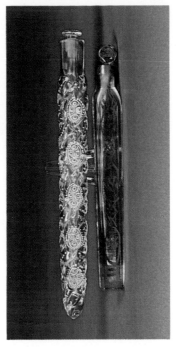

Lot #120. Pair of 19th century clear glass 'lavender' bottles and stoppers, 7.1" [18 cm] and 5.6" [14.2 cm], the longer bottle molded with swirls and enameled in white, blue, yellow and red, smaller bottle enameled in gold. Two items. Est. $75.00-$150.00.

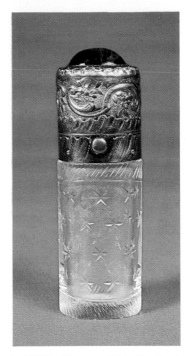

Lot #121. Clear crystal bottle of cylinder form with silver gilt mount, 3.2" [8.1 cm], the body of the bottle decorated with stars, the hinged metal top mounted with a large green stone surrounded by smaller clear ones [tiny flake on bottom], back of metal fitting bearing a small loop. Est. $175.00-$250.00.

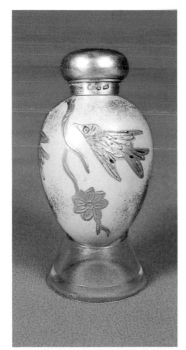

Lot #122. Ceramic scent bottle shaped as an egg, with sterling silver top, 2.5" [6.4 cm], the body of the bottle painted a delicate light green, and decorated with birds in flight in gold and silver, the sterling silver fittings with English hallmarks for Birmingham, 1912. Est. $400.00-$500.00.

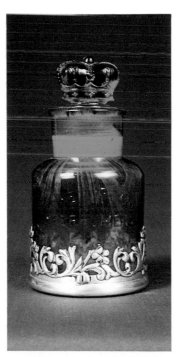

Lot #123. The Crown Perfumery green glass bottle and stopper, 5" [12.7 cm], the bottle of apothecary form with a crown stopper, empty, name molded onto side of bottle, in a silver holder with a design registry mark from 1898. Est. $75.00-$150.00.

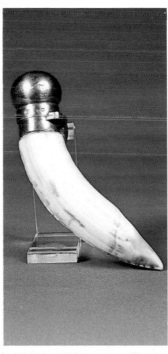

Lot #124. 19th century English carved horn perfume bottle, 4.6" [11.7 cm], curved shape, intricate mount of sterling silver which must be turned to allow it to open, English hallmarks for London, 1881. Est. $125.00-$175.00.

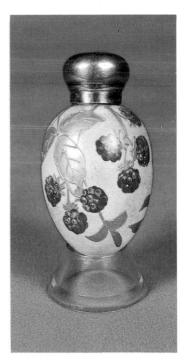

Lot #125. Ceramic scent bottle shaped as an egg, with sterling silver top, 2.5" [6.4 cm], the body of the bottle painted in shades of pink against which there are handpainted black raspberries and gold leaves; neck stamped with English hallmarks for Birmingham, 1912, bottom with a design registry mark for 1885. Est. $400.00-$500.00.

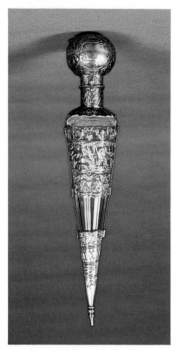

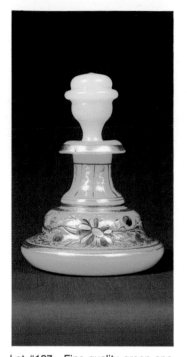

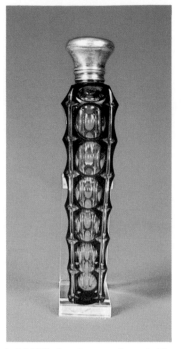

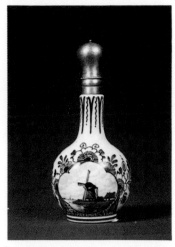

Lot #126. Elaborate clear crystal bottle of parasol shape with continental silver filigree mount and cap, 9" [22.9 cm], most of the body of the bottle covered with a silver metal frieze of scenes with people and animals, hinged ball top with inner stopper, unmarked. Est. $350.00-$400.00.

Lot #127. Fine quality green opaline glass perfume bottle and stopper, 5" [12.7 cm], a beautiful design typical of the late 19th century, almost a bell-form, the exterior decorated with flowers in gold, blue, and brown enamel, polished bottom, maker unidentified. Est. $300.00-$400.00.

Lot #128. Laydown perfume bottle of clear crystal overlaid with blue, 5" [12.7 cm], the body of the bottle with four sides cut with oval windows of graduated sizes, silver metal top with glass inner stopper; probably of Bohemian manufacture. Est. $200.00-$300.00.

Lot #129. Delft fine quality porcelain bottle with silver cap and inner stopper, 4" [10.2 cm], beautifully hand-painted with a windmill scene and floral motifs, bottom signed *Delft De Porceleyne Fles*, numbered, and with artist's initials. Est. $150.00-$250.00.

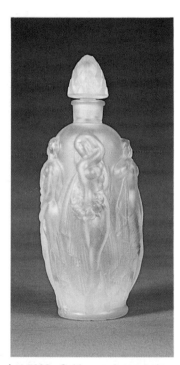

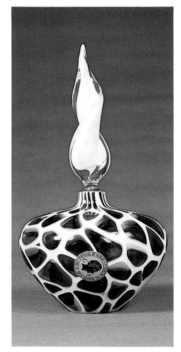

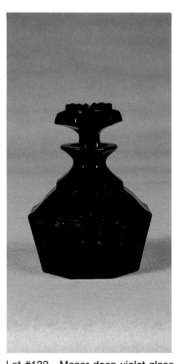

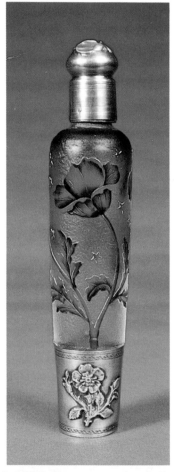

Lot #130. Sabino opalescent glass bottle and stopper, 6.1" [15.5 cm], the slender form of the bottle entirely covered by a continuous panel of thinly clad women with garlands of flowers, stopper with a diamond motif, signed Sabino in script and with red and gold paper label. Est. $150.00-$200.00.

Lot #131. Italian mosaic glass bottle and white and clear cased glass stopper, 6.9" [17.5 cm], the mosaic stones of red, blue, and green in a background of white, stopper molded as a flame, with gold label on side marked Murano Italy. Est. $75.00-$125.00.

Lot #132. Moser deep violet glass bottle and stopper, 3" [7.6 cm], of faceted inkwell shape with eight sides, stopper also molded with a pinwheel design, bottom signed in acid Moser Bohemia. Est. $250.00-$300.00.

Lot #133. Daum cameo glass bottle of frosted clear and light blue glass, 6" [15.2 cm], the bottle cut with a design of oriental poppies highlighted in black and gold enamel, silver base and cap with conforming flower motifs, cap hallmarked, base signed in gold enamel Daum Nancy and the *Croix de Lorraine*. Est. $900.00-$1000.00.

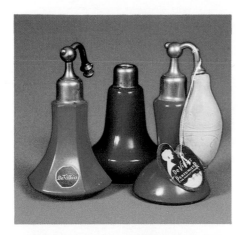

Lot #134. Lot of three small DeVilbiss atomizers, tallest 4.3" [10.9 cm], each of clear glass enameled in pink, two with DeVilbiss tags, one with bulb lacking, one with atomizer lacking. Three items. Est. $75.00-$125.00.

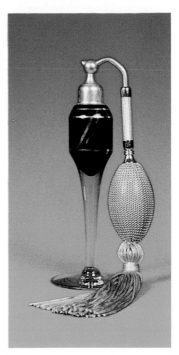

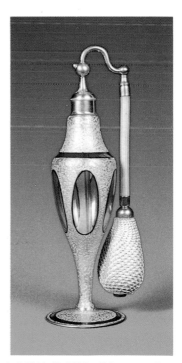

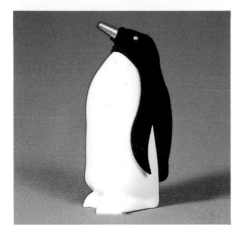

Lot #135. Lenox porcelain penguin with atomizer made for DeVilbiss, 4.4" [11.2 cm], the black felt cape conceals the atomizer bulb and the sprayer is the penguin's nose, bottom signed DeVilbiss in green enamel and Lenox USA. Est. $200.00-$300.00.

Lot #136. DeVilbiss amber and black cased glass dropper perfume bottle, 7" [17.8 cm], gold enamel decor, stopper with dauber, glass probably by the Cambridge Glass Co., unsigned. Est. $200.00-$300.00.

Lot #137. American clear glass atomizer, 6.6" [16.8 cm], the well internally decorated in black, the exterior with a design in gold enamel, functioning atomizer, maker unidentified. Est. $150.00-$200.00.

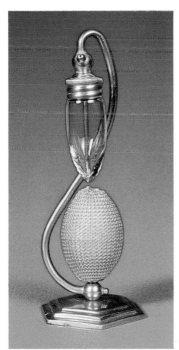

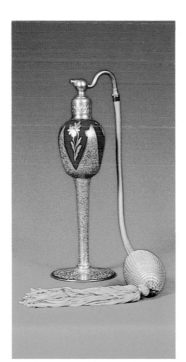

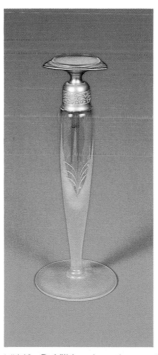

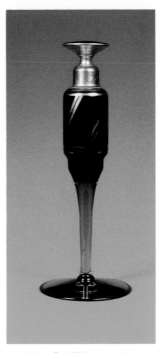

Lot #138. DeVilbiss light pink glass perfume bottle atomizer, 5.9" [15 cm], mounted in an elaborate Art Deco style holder with curving brass and hexagonal base, functioning gold atomizer ball, bottom marked "Patent Allowed." Est. $275.00-$400.00.

Lot #139. Pyramid clear glass bottle internally decorated in blue, the exterior acid-etched and decorated in gold, 7.4" [18.8 cm], neck hardware marked Pyramid, functioning atomizer bulb and tassel. Est. $300.00-$400.00.

Lot #140. DeVilbiss clear glass and frosted light blue dropper bottle, 6.5" [16.5 cm], sides of the bottle wheel cut with a leaf design, metal stopper with long dauber and light blue glass medallion on top, bottom signed DeVilbiss. Est. $400.00-$500.00.

Lot #141. DeVilbiss light green glass atomizer bottle, 8" [20.3 cm], the bottle decorated with oval windows outlined in black, the rest of the bottle heavily acid-etched and covered in gold enamel, hardware marked DeVilbiss, original atomizer bulb [hard], bottom signed DeVilbiss. Est. $350.00-$450.00.

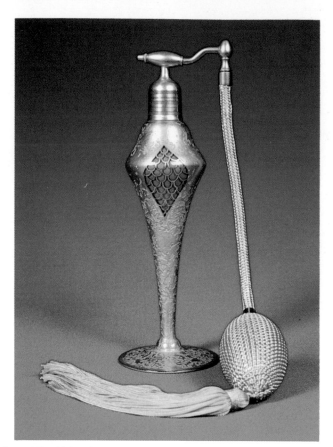

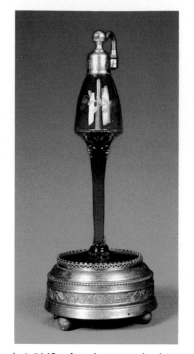

Lot #143. American peach glass atomizer bottle mounted on a music box, total height 9" [22.9 cm], the bottle wheel cut with a band of flowers [bulb lacking]. Est. $300.00-$400.00.

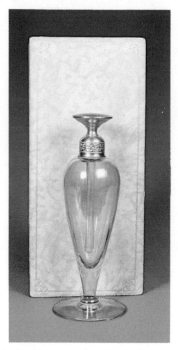

Lot #144. Fine quality DeVilbiss perfume bottle, 6.2" [15.7 cm], the bottle of inverted teardrop shape in a delicate caramel iridescent color, stopper with long dauber enameled black and gold, bottom acid etched DeVilbiss, in its original presentation case with satin interior; box with DeVilbiss sticker. Est. $300.00-$400.00.

Lot #142. Volupté glass atomizer bottle, 7" [17.8 cm], the well internally decorated in green, the exterior heavily acid-etched and with three windows decorated with a fishscale motif, functioning atomizer, label on base "22 kt gold plated decorated." Est. $300.00-$450.00.

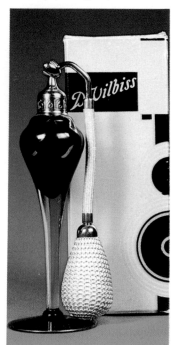

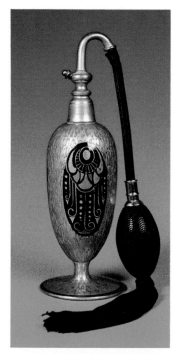

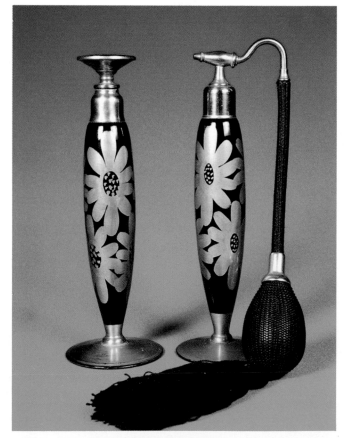

Lot #145. DeVilbiss clear glass atomizer bottle internally decorated in black and with silver enamel decoration of the exterior, 6.5" [16.5 cm], all original silver atomizer fittings [ball hardened], unsigned, in its original green and black box with model #S48-5 on bottom. Est. $250.00-$350.00.

Lot #146. French black glass atomizer bottle, 7.7" [19.5 cm], the egg-shaped well heavily acid-etched and decorated with three oval medallions each with beautiful Art Deco motifs, [replaced atomizer ball and tassel], hardware marked France. Est. $450.00-$600.00. This is quite possibly the type of elegant and beautiful bottle that was seen by Thomas DeVilbiss and Frédéric Vuillemenot at the 1925 Paris Exposition.

Lot #147. Pair of American black glass atomizer and dropper bottles, 7" [17.8 cm], each of cigar form, both elaborately decorated in gold enamel with flowers [some wear to gold on base of dropper bottle], functioning atomizer, maker unidentified. Two bottles. Est. $450.00-$600.00.

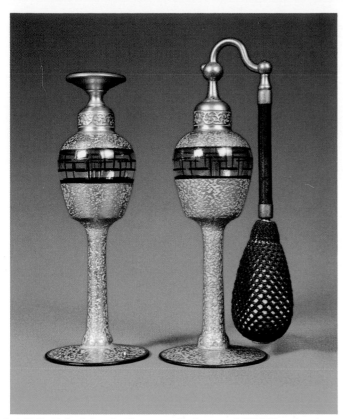

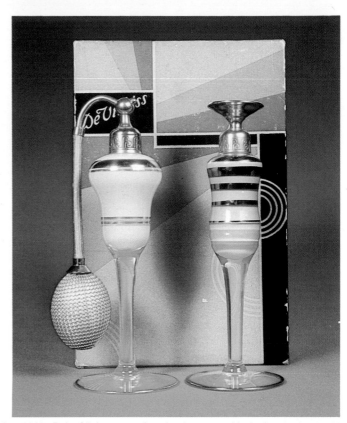

Lot #148. Pair of glass bottles, one with dropper, 6.2" [15.7 cm], and one with atomizer, 7" [17.8 cm], each with a clear band decorated in black enamel, exterior etched and enameled gold, all original [hard ball], each signed DeVilbiss in gold enamel. 2 items. Est. $150.00-$600.00.

Lot #149. Pair of light green glass bottles, one with dauber and one with atomizer, both 6.4" [16.3 cm], the exterior decorated with gold rings, possibly by Cambridge Glass Co., unsigned, unused condition, in their green, silver, and black Art Deco box marked DeVilbiss. Est. $450.00-$500.00.

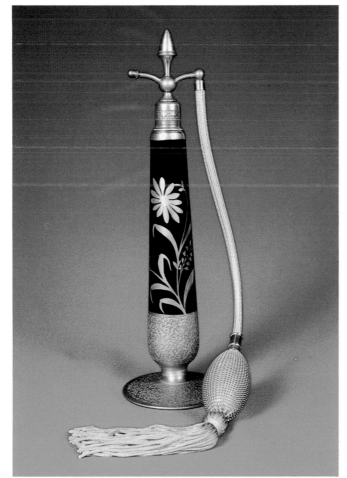

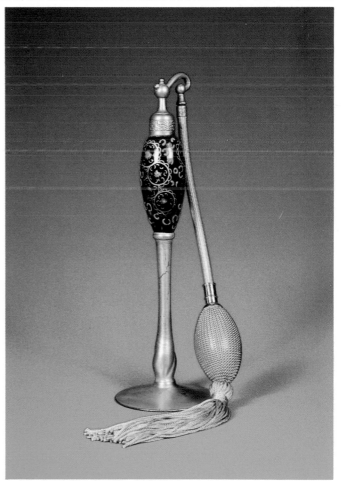

Lot #150. DeVilbiss statuesque black glass atomizer bottle, 10.7" [27 cm], with flowers in gold enamel, the base acid-etched and enameled in gold, unsigned, DeVilbiss 'acorn' on hardware. Est. $600.00-$750.00.

Lot #151. DeVilbiss extremely tall clear and satinized glass atomizer bottle, 9.5" [24.1 cm], the exterior enameled in coral and gold, very minor wear to gold, signed DeVilbiss. Est. $500.00-$650.00.

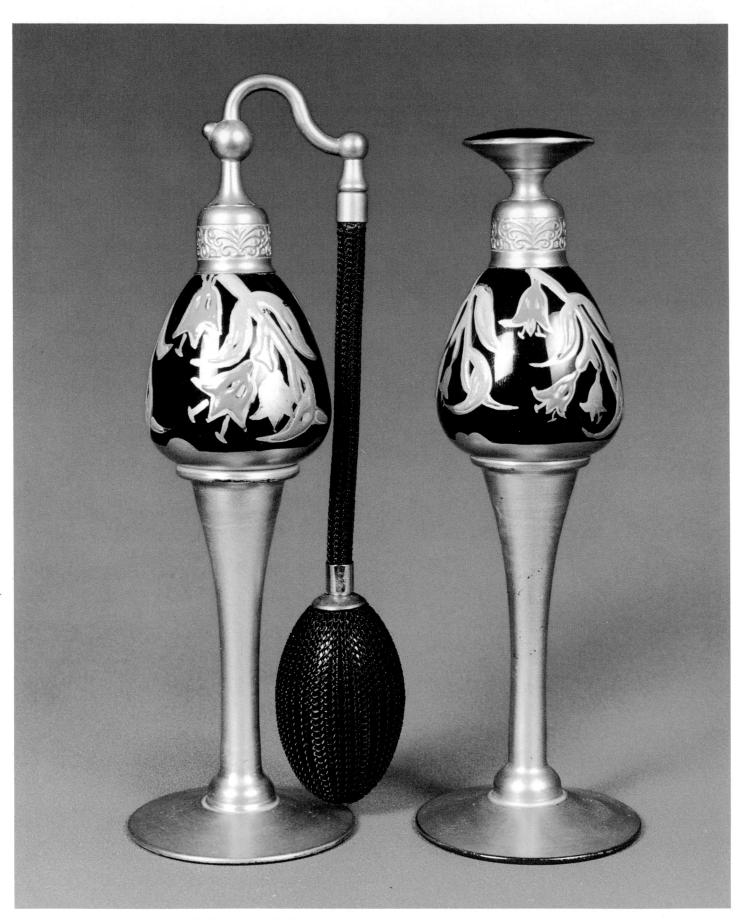

Lot #152. Pair of DeVilbiss glass bottles, one with dropper 7" [17.8 cm], one with atomizer, 7.5" [19 cm], the wells decorated in black enamel and with flowers and leaves in orange and green [tiny enamel restoration on one], the pedestals decorated in gold, both signed DeVilbiss on base. Est. $800.00-$1000.00.

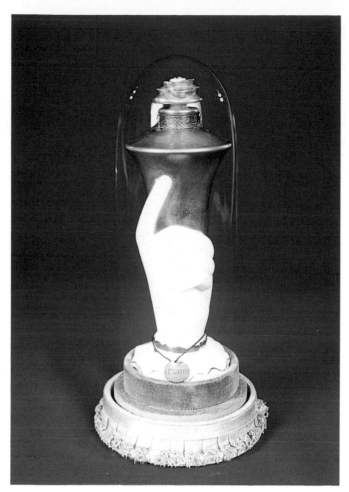

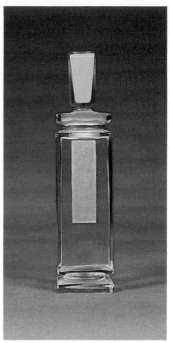

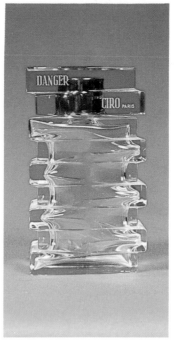

Lot #153. Elizabeth Arden *It's You* white crystal bottle and stopper, 6.3" [16 cm], modeled as a hand holding a vase with rose stopper, empty, vase and stopper enameled in gold, Baccarat emblem on bottom, apparently empty but unopened, metal tag label around wrist, in its original dome marked France. Bacc #781 [1939]. Est. $2500.00-$3000.00.

Lot #154. Caron *Les Pois de Senteur de Chez Moi* ['My Own Sweet Peas'], clear crystal bottle and stopper, 6" [15.2 cm], an elegant rectangular form on a footed base, stopper with green enamel, label, empty, inside Baccarat emblem on bottom. Bacc #809 [1947]. Est. $100.00-$200.00.

Lot #155. Ciro *Danger* unusual clear crystal bottle, inner stopper, and massive overcap, 4.1" [10.5 cm], a geometric Art Deco design with stacked rectangles, empty, names in gold enamel on overcap, inside of overcap also enameled in gold, Baccarat emblem on base; this is possibly a special edition, since the overcap is not black. Bacc. #777 [1938]. Est. $350.00-$450.00.

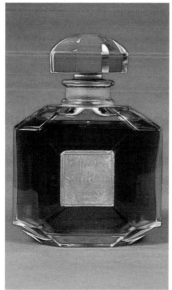

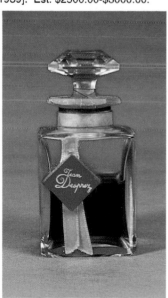

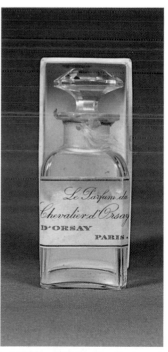

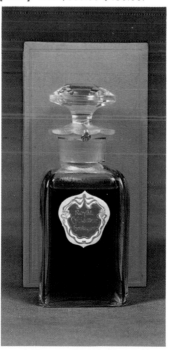

Lot #156. Corday *Le Pois de Senteur* clear crystal bottle and stopper, 4.8" [12.2 cm], the bottle of irregular octagonal form with faceted edges, the stopper also octagonal and with rounded facets, central groove to tie stopper, full, label, bottom with Baccarat emblem. Bacc #590 [1925-34]. Est. $150.00-$250.00.

Lot #157. Jean Desprez *Etourdissant* ['Stunning'] clear crystal bottle and stopper, 3.7" [9.5 cm], of rectangular decanter form, with perfume and sealed, label is a pink leather medallion on front, Baccarat emblem and label on base. Bacc. #111 [1911 and later]. Est. $200.00-$275.00.

Lot #158. D'Orsay *Le Parfum du Chevalier d'Orsay* clear crystal bottle and stopper, 4" [10.2 cm], the bottle of decanter shape, empty, label across the front of the bottle, bottom of box only, Baccarat emblem on base; this is the very early namesake perfume of this famous company. Bacc. #10 [1912 for D'Orsay]. Est. $150.00-$250.00.

Lot #159. Houbigant *Royal Cyclamen* clear crystal bottle and stopper, 4.1" [10.4 cm], of decanter shape, stopper molded with facets, full and sealed, Baccarat emblem on base, in its box of deep pink. Bacc. #10 [1907-1923 for Houbigant]. Est. $200.00-$300.00.

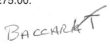
BACCARAT

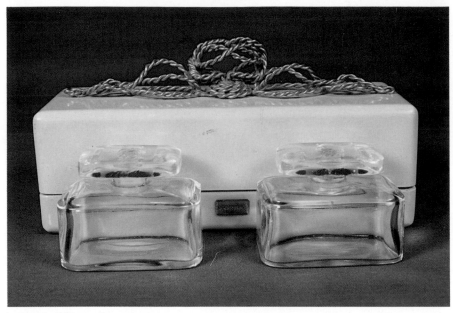

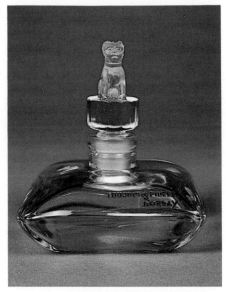

Lot #160. D'Orsay *Duo* pair of clear crystal bottles and stoppers, 1.7" (4.3 cm), of short rectangular form with stoppers of conforming shape, the portrait of the Count d'Orsay in 19th century attire molded into the stopper, empty, unsigned, in their unusual wood box with D'Orsay metal tag and elaborate wire decoration. Bacc. #793 [1944]. Est. $300.00-$400.00.

Lot #161. D'Orsay *Toujours Fidèle* ['Always Faithful'] clear crystal bottle and stopper, 3.5" [8.9 cm], of pillow form, empty, names enameled in black on front, stopper molded with a sitting dog, amber patina, unsigned. Bacc. #162 [1912]. Est. $275.00-$350.00.

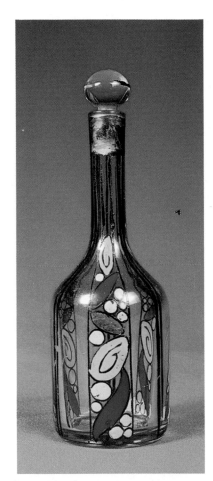

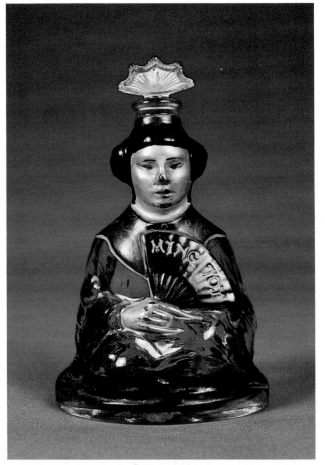

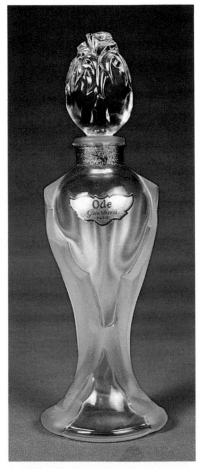

Lot #162. D'Hortys [fragrance unidentified] clear crystal bottle and stopper, 5.1" [13 cm], in the shape of a miniature wine bottle with ball stopper, the sides enameled in pink, blue, green, and yellow with a very early modernistic, abstract design [some wear to enamel], Baccarat emblem on bottom. Bacc. #359 [1917] Est. $300.00-$400.00.

Lot #163. Forest *Ming Toy* very rare clear crystal bottle and stopper, 4.3" [11 cm], in the shape of an oriental lady seated and holding a fan with the words Ming Toy, beautifully enameled in blue, black, and gold, with some perfume, stopper frozen, some wear to enamel, bottom with Baccarat emblem. Bacc. #510 [1923]. Cf. Lefkowith, p. 125, #100. Est. $2500.00-$3500.00.

Lot #164. Guerlain *Ode* very large clear crystal bottle and stopper, 7.3" [18.5 cm], the stopper molded as a complete rosebud, the base with graceful curvilinear design and part frosted, empty, gold label, Baccarat emblem on bottom. Bacc. #816 [1954]. Est. $350.00-$450.00.

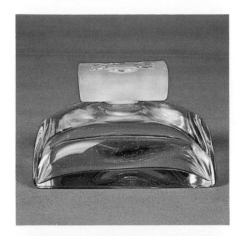

Lot #165. D'Orsay *La Trophée* clear crystal bottle and frosted glass stopper, 1.6" [4 cm], of unusual inkwell form, the frosted stopper impressed with the coat of arms of the Count d'Orsay, empty, Baccarat emblem on bottom. Bacc. #757 [1935]. Est. $250.00-$325.00.

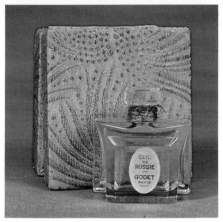

Lot #166. Godet *Cuir de Russie* ['Russian Leather'] clear crystal bottle and stopper, 2.1" [5.3 cm], the bottle sculpted as a beautiful geometric form, empty, gold label on front, Baccarat seal on base, in its box [interior stains] covered with lavender and silver brocade. Bacc. #762 [1936]. Est. $500.00-$600.00.

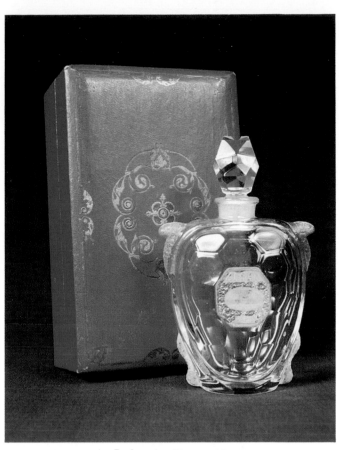

Lot #167. Guerlain *Le Parfum des Champs Élysees*, rare clear crystal bottle and stopper, 4.5" [11.4 cm], molded in the form of a turtle, the arms and feet of the turtle frosted and patinated gray, empty, label on front is quite worn, Baccarat emblem on base, in its seldom seen red box with cream silk interior. Bacc. #284 [1914]. Cf. Lefkowith, p. 93, #87. Est. $1000.00-$1200.00.

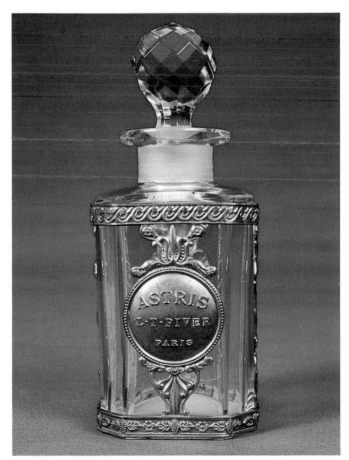

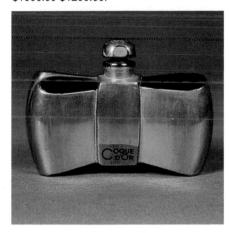

Lot #169. Guerlain *Coq d'Or* cobalt crystal bottle and stopper in the form of a bowtie, 2.1" [5.3 cm], covered in gold enamel, names in black enamel on either side, Baccarat emblem on bottom. Bacc. #770 [1937]. Est. $400.00-$500.00.

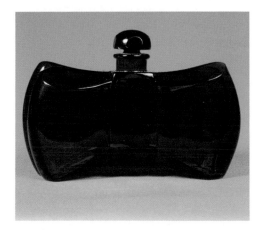

Lot #170. Guerlain *Coq d'Or* or *Dawamesk* huge size blue crystal bottle and stopper in the form of a bowtie, 4" tall by 5.8" wide [10.2 x 14.7 cm], Guerlain and Baccarat emblems on bottom. Bacc. #770 [1937]. This large size is uncommon. Est. $500.00-$600.00.

Lot #168. L. T. Piver *Astris* [Latin: 'To the Stars'] clear crystal bottle and stopper, 4.7" [12 cm], the bottle of decanter shape with faceted corners, the stopper a faceted ball, the entire bottle encased in a metal frame bearing the label on front, numbered stopper, unsigned. Bacc. #398 [1919]. Est. $350.00-$450.00.

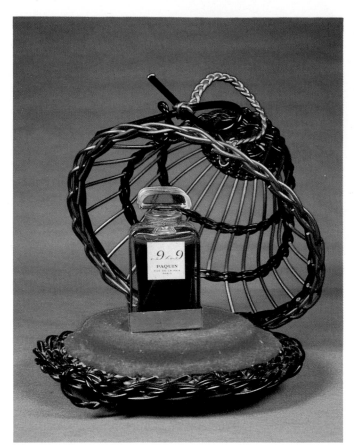

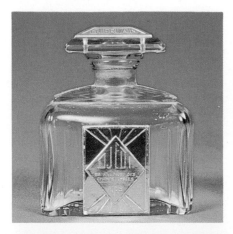

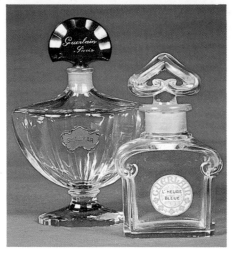

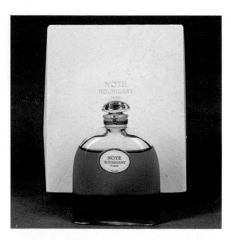

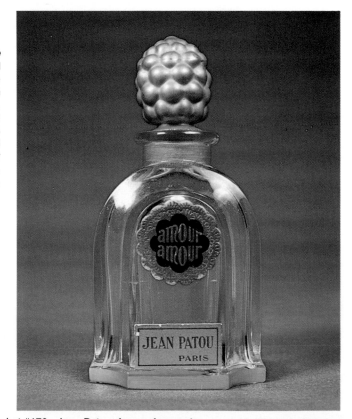

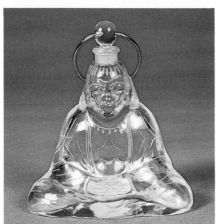

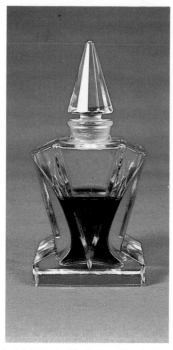

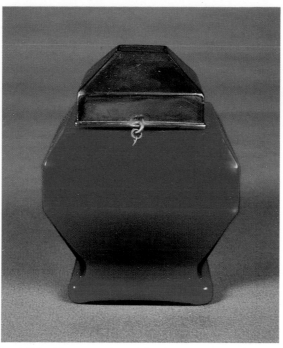

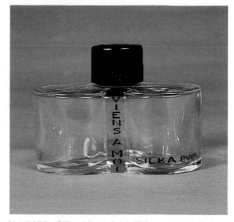

Lot #179. Silka *Viens à Moi* ['Come to Me'] clear crystal bottle, inner stopper and overcap, 2.8" [7.1 cm], the bottle designed with two round sections resembling a figure 8, silver metal collar around neck, wooden overcap with an age fracture, names enameled on front in black, empty, Baccarat emblem on base. Bacc. #712 [1930]. Est. $400.00-$500.00.

Lot #177. L. M. B. C., Elbeuf clear crystal bottle and stopper, 4.3" [11 cm], the bottle with an unusual "V" design, faceted pointed stopper, some perfume, Baccarat emblem on bottom. Bacc. #795 [1945]. Est. $200.00 $300.00.

Lot #178. Myon cased crystal red over white bottle, inner stopper, and brass metal overcap with red enamel medallion, 3.5" [8.9 cm], empty, metal tag label lacking, bottom with Baccarat emblem and signed in acid Myon. Bacc. #667 [1928]. Est. $700.00-$850.00.

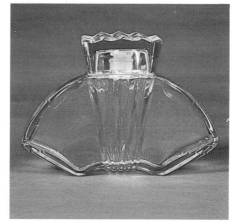

Lot #180. Verlayne *Attente* clear crystal perfume bottle, stopper, and overcap, 3.3" (8.3 cm), in the shape of a fan, Baccarat emblem on base. Bacc. #803 [1946]. Est. $200.00-$300.00.

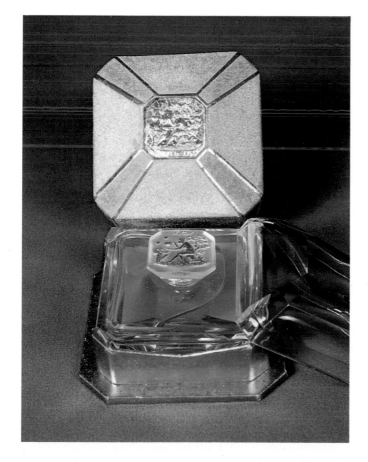

Lot #181. Molinelle *Gardenia* special edition rare crystal bottle, inner stopper, and glass overcap, 1.9" [4.8 cm], the stopper designed with the goddess Aphrodite blowing heart shaped bubbles from a bowl held by Eros, full and sealed, the "dauber" is a string of glass beads, crystal probably of Czechoslovakian manufacture, in its seldom seen box. Cf. Lefkowith, p. 159, #172-174. Est. $1000.00-$1200.00.

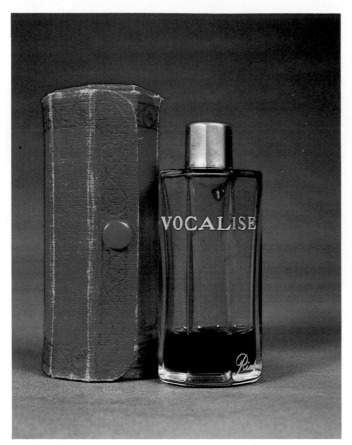

Lot #182. Rimmel *Vocalise* clear crystal bottle, inner stopper, and overcap, 3.2" [8 cm], the bottle of octagonal column form, some perfume, names in gold enamel in inset letters, in its silk lined red box [worn], signed Baccarat on base. Bacc. #522 [1923]. Est. $500.00-$600.00.

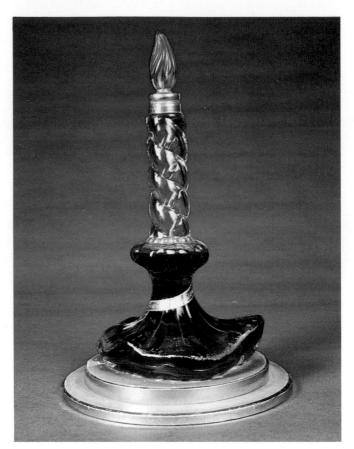

Lot #183. Schiaparelli *Sleeping* huge size clear crystal bottle and red crystal stopper, 8" [20.3 cm], molded in the shape of a candle decorated with gold, with perfume, label around candle, Baccarat emblem on base, with original blue plinth. Bacc #778 [1939]. Est. $500.00-$650.00.

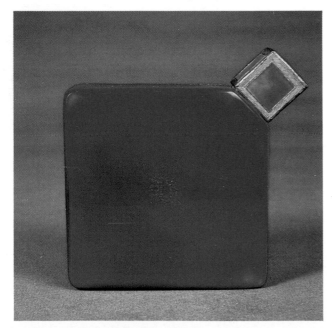

Lot #184. Ybry *Désir du Coeur* ['Heart's Desire'] red over white cased crystal bottle and stopper, 3.1" [7.9 cm] to top of stopper, metal overcap in pink enamel and inner stopper, empty, [label lacking], base signed with Baccarat emblem. Bacc #583 [1925-1927]. Est. $600.00-$750.00.

COMMERCIAL PERFUME BOTTLES

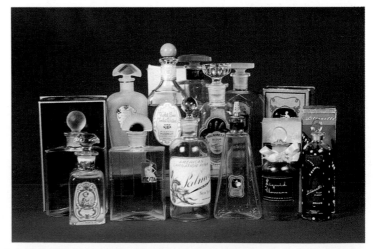

Lot #185. Perfume history - lot of twelve late 19th century and 20th century cologne bottles, some with boxes: Baldwin (Chicago) *Queen Bess;* Foote & Jenks (Jackson, Michigan) *Mignonette;* Palmer *American Carnation* and *Fiesta;* Harmony (Boston) *Bouquet Ramée;* Richard Hudnut *Arbutus, Three Flowers, Violet Sec;* Massenet *Altesse;* Parkinson *Liquid Flowers;* Pinaud *Lilianelli;* Stearns *Pompadour* [stopper frozen]. Twelve items. Est. $120.00-$240.00.

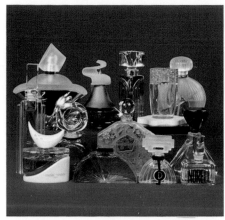

Lot #186. Lot of 13 contemporary designer perfumes, heights from 1.9" to 6.1" [4.8 to 15.5 cm], some factice: Lagerfeld *KL;* Norell; Parfums International *Decadence;* Nina Ricci *Nina;* Bijan; Jean-Louis Scherrer *2;* Marc Sinan *Sinan;* Houbigant *Raffinée;* Romeo Gigli; Brosseau *Ombre Rose;* Herb Alpert *Listen;* Liz Claiborne; Shulton *Escapade.* Thirteen items. Est. $120.00-$240.00.

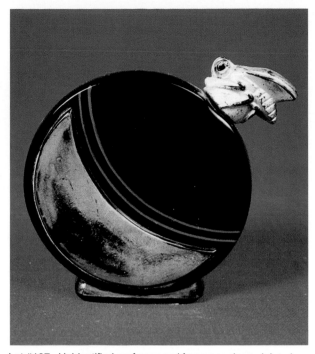

Lot #187. Unidentified perfumer and fragrance deep violet glass [appearing as black] bottle and composition cap in the form of a bee, 3.8" [9.7 cm], the circular bottle molded with a crescent moon in silver [worn] and lines in red enamel, bee enameled silver and with red dots, no label. Est. $450.00-$600.00.

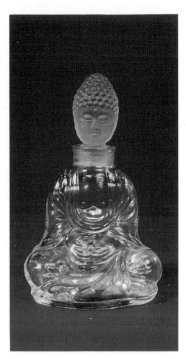

Lot #188. Unidentified clear glass bottle with frosted glass stopper, 3.7" [9.4 cm], the entirety molded as a sitting Buddha with hands in symbolic pose, head with amber patina, empty, no labels [small chip on lip, tongue of stopper with small chips]; similar to many made for Vantine's. Est. $125.00-$200.00.

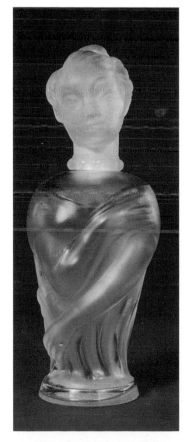

Lot #189. Elizabeth Arden *Mémoire Chérie* very large size frosted glass bottle and inner stopper [chip on inner stopper] and overcap in the form of a woman, 7" [17.8 cm], bottom molded Arden Made in France, empty, large gold label on bottom. Est. $600.00-$750.00.

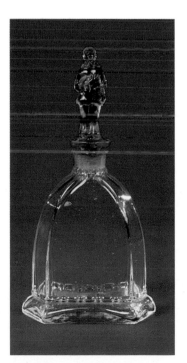

Lot #190. Unidentified perfume and perfumer, clear glass bottle and turquoise glass stopper, 5.1" [13 cm], the stopper molded as a standing Pierrot. Est. $300.00-$400.00.

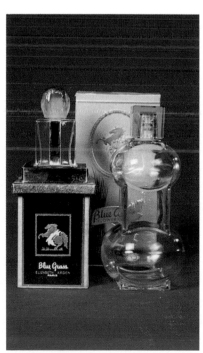

Lot #191. Elizabeth Arden *Blue Grass* clear glass bottle and inner stopper with turquoise blue overcap molded with mare and colt, 2.7" [6.9 cm], empty, blue and silver label, traces of gold enamel on the overcap, in its blue and gold box and outer box; *Blue Grass* cologne clear glass bottle and turquoise glass cap, 5.9" [15 cm], empty, no label, in its blue box. Two items. Est. $250.00-$300.00.

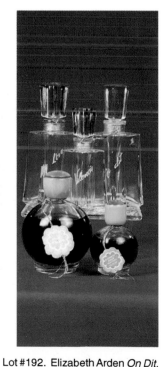

Lot #192. Elizabeth Arden *On Dit, My Love,* and *Valencia* clear glass bottles + stoppers, 4.5" [11.5 cm] and 3.7" [9.5 cm], all empty; *Mille Fleurs* [2] ball-shaped bottles, glass inner stoppers and bakelite overcaps, 3.3" [8.5 cm] and 2.6" [6.5 cm], full and sealed, labels at neck and on bottom. Five items. Est. $150.00-$300.00.

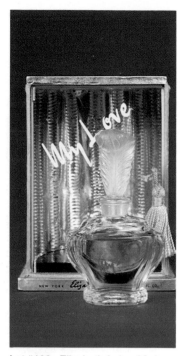

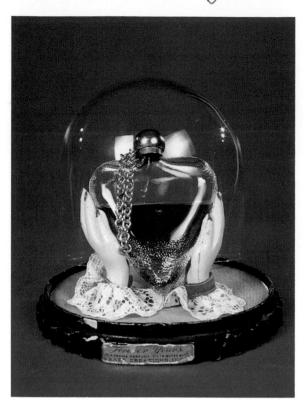

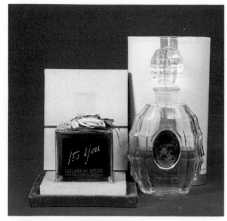

Lot #195. Elizabeth Arden *It's You* clear glass bottle and stopper, 3.1" [8 cm], both bottle and stopper in the form of perfect cubes, full and sealed, flowers and ribbon at neck, purple foil label, in its box; clear glass bottle and stopper with quilted motif for cologne, 5.4" [13.7 cm], in its pink box. Two items. Est. $100.00-$150.00.

Lot #193. Elizabeth Arden *My Love* clear glass bottle and frosted glass stopper, 3.4" [8.6 cm], stopper molded in the form of a feather, name in gold enamel on front, some perfume, in its gold foil box with lucite door and tassel. Cf. Lefkowith, p. 175, #198. Est. $400.00-$500.00.

Lot #194. Babs Creations *Forever Yours* clear glass bottle and brass ball cap with a chain, 3" [7.6 cm], shaped as a heart, some perfume, held by two metal hands under a glass dome, gold label at bottom of metal holder. Est. $150.00-$250.00.

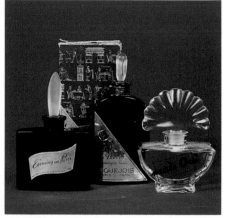

Lot #196. Bourjois *Soir de Paris* blue glass bottle with frosted glass stopper, 4.5" [11.4 cm], near full and sealed, silver label, in its blue and silver box; *Evening in Paris* blue glass bottle and frosted glass stopper, 3.9" [10 cm], silver label, empty; *Mais Oui* ['But Yes'] clear glass bottle and stopper, 3.4" [8.6 cm], black enamel label, empty. 3 items. Est. $200.00-$300.00.

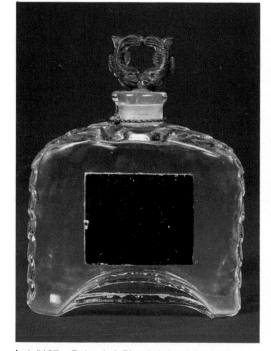

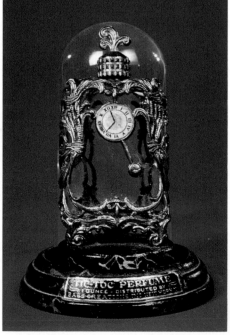

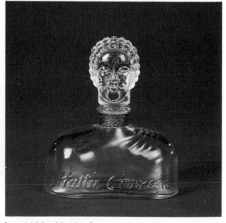

Lot #197. Babani *A Blend* clear glass bottle and frosted glass stopper in the form of two dolphins whose heads and tails meet, 3.2" [8.1 cm], age-darkened label also reads "A Perfume from Elizabeth Arden" [...who distributed Babani in the USA], bottom also molded Babani Paris. Est. $400.00-$500.00.

Lot #198. Babs *Tic Toc* Perfume clear glass bottle and metal screw-on stopper in the shape of a clock fitted on a base with glass dome, total height 5.2" [13.2 cm], label on front of base, empty. Est. $125.00-$175.00.

Lot #199. Hattie Carnegie *Carnegie Pink* medium size clear glass bottle and stopper, 3.4" [8.6 cm], in the shape of a woman's head and shoulders in Art Deco style, name spelled out in raised letters at bottom; label on bottom, empty. Est. $200.00-$250.00.

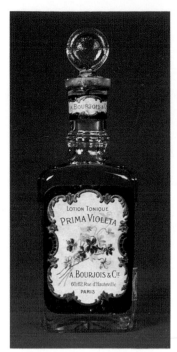

Lot #200. Bourjois *Prima Violeta* clear glass bottle and stopper, 7.9" [20 cm], of antique shape often used in the late 19th century, full and sealed, labels around neck, on front, with special Bourjois label on side, reverse of bottle molded with Bourjois name and logo, overall unusually fine condition considering its age. Est. $75.00-$150.00.

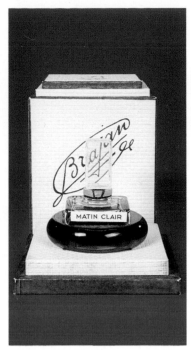

Lot #201. Brajan *Matin Clair* ['Clear Morning'] clear glass bottle and stopper, 2.5" [6.4 cm], the bottle an interesting Art Deco geometric design of stacked squares and circle, full and sealed, label on front, in its original box. Est. $175.00 $225.00.

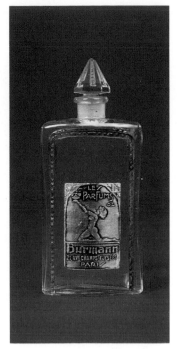

Lot #202. Burmann *Les Parfums de Burmann* clear glass bottle and stopper, 4.2" [10.7 cm], both bottle and stopper molded with an inset border of beads which are patinated gray, empty, beautiful silver label showing an Art Deco nude holding a perfume lamp. Est. $250.00-$300.00.

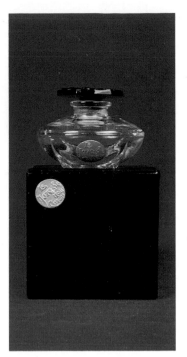

Lot #203. Caron *Le Narcisse Noir* clear glass bottle and black glass stopper, 2" [5.1 cm], the bottle of round, flattened shape, stopper in the form of a narcissus fully opened, empty, gold label on side of bottle, in its black box. Est. $100.00-$150.00.

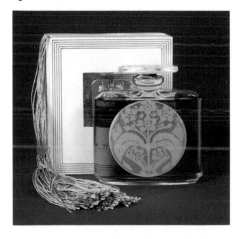

Lot #204. Caron *Le Tabac Blond* ['White Tobacco'] clear glass bottle and stopper, 3.3" [8.4 cm], the bottle of flat oval shape, stopper molded with Caron and frosted, gold label of a tobacco flower on front, label also on base, full and sealed, in its tasseled book-form box and outer box. Est. $150.00-$250.00.

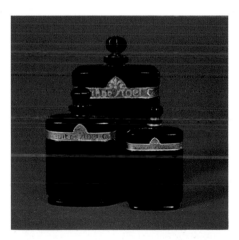

Lot #205. Caron *Nuit de Noël* black glass bottles and stoppers, three graduated sizes, 4.3", 3.1", 2.8" [11 cm, 8 cm, 7 cm], of flask shape with ball stoppers, silver labels around bottles, empty. Three items. Est. $100.00-$125.00.

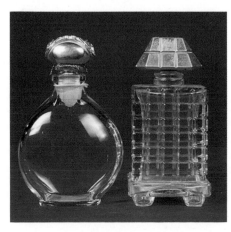

Lot #206. Caron *Or et Noir* ['Gold and Black'] clear glass bottle and stopper, 4.1 " [10.4 cm], the stopper molded with two bees and covered in gold, empty, label on bottom; *La Fête des Roses* ['A Celebration of Roses'] clear glass bottle and stopper, 4.1" [10.4 cm], the rectangular form with cross-hatched lines, stopper enameled in gold, empty, label on bottom. Two items. Est. $300.00-$400.00.

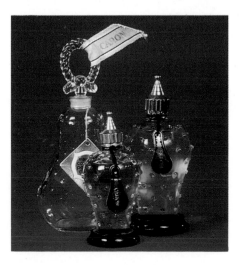

Lot #207. Caron *Poivre* ['Pepper'] lot of three bottles: clear glass bottle and stopper of pear shape, 6.8" [17.3 cm], stopper shaped as a loop of rope, label around neck and on stopper, empty; two clear glass bottles with metal caps, 5.5" and 4.5" [14 cm and 11 cm], decorated with rows of dots, full, labels around neck. Three items. Est. $150.00-$225.00.

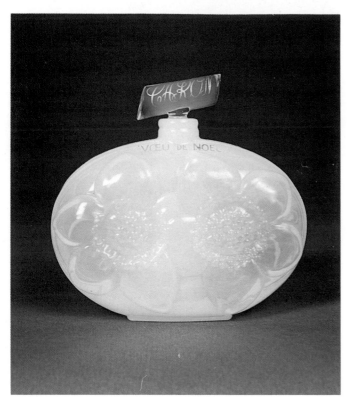

Lot #208. Caron *Voeu de Noel* opalescent white glass bottle and stopper, 3.6" [9.1 cm], empty, the front molded with a pair of open flowers, the stopper as a small bar, name and company enameled perfectly in gold on front, bottom acid marked France. Est. $600.00-$750.00.

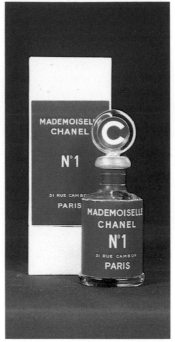

Lot #209. Chanel *No. 1* rare and important clear glass bottle and stopper of antique apothecary shape, 4.1" [10.5 cm], red and white label around most of bottle and neck, label readss: Mademoiselle Chanel, 31, rue Cambon, "C" label also on stopper, bottom molded Mademoiselle Chanel Paris France, sealed with some perfume, in a cream colored box. Est. $600.00-$800.00.

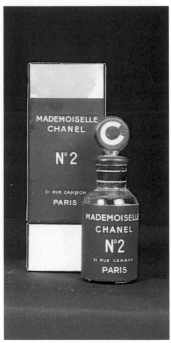

Lot #210. Chanel *No. 2* rare clear glass bottle and stopper of antique apothecary shape, 3.9" [10 cm], red and white label around most of bottle and neck, label states: Mademoiselle Chanel, 31, rue Cambon, "C" label also on stopper, sealed but perfume evaporated, in a cream colored box with perfume stains; slight differences between this bottle and that of *No.1*. Est. $500.00-$700.00.

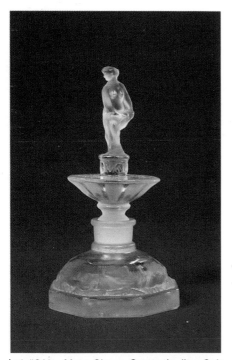

Lot #211. Mary Chess *Souvenir d'un Soir* ['Memory of an Evening'] clear and frosted bottle and stopper, 3.5" [8.9 cm], molded as a miniature replica of the fountain outside the Plaza Hotel in New York, empty. Est. $600.00-$750.00.

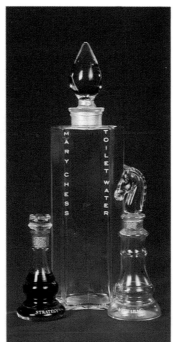

Lot #212. Mary Chess *White Lilac* clear glass bottle and stopper, 4.4" [11.2 cm], a knight, empty, name in white enamel; *Strategy* clear glass bottle and stopper, 2.9" [7.4 cm], a castle, name in white enamel, full and sealed; *Toilet Water* clear glass bottle and stopper shaped like a star, 7.9" [20 cm], empty, name in white. Three items. Est. $175.00-$250.00.

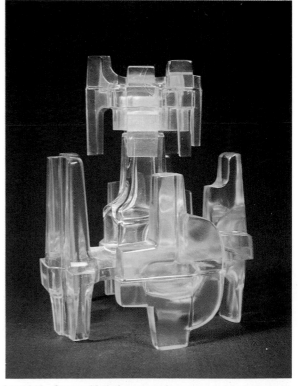

Lot #213. Carven *Variations* rare clear glass bottle and plastic cap, 4.6" [11.7 cm], the bottle of unusual abstract shape, fitted into a holder of yellow plastic which forms an artistic unity with the bottle and stopper, molded label on top, marked *Sculpté par Mannoni*, empty. Est. $250.00-$350.00.

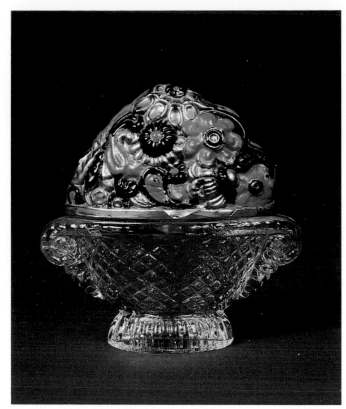

Lot #214. Corday *Serre Fleurie* ['Hothouse Blossoms'], clear glass bottle, inner stopper and heavy glass overcap, 4.4" [11.2 cm], the bottle molded as a basket or urn [there is a hole in the glass on one corner], the overcap as a mass of highly stylized blossoms enameled in orange, gold, and black; circa 1924, it was expensive at the time and the bottle is quite rare today. Est. $200.00-$300.00.

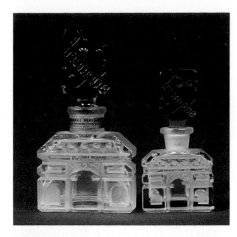

Lot #215. Carrel *Triomphe* pair of clear and frosted glass bottles, one with green stopper, 3.6" [9.1 cm], one with red stopper, 2.8" [7.1 cm], each molded in the form of the Arc de Triomphe, name molded into stoppers, empty, larger one with label around neck. Two items. Est. $200.00-$275.00.

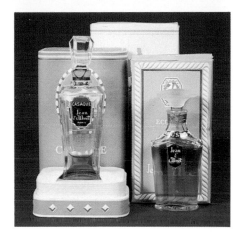

Lot #216. Jean d'Albret *Casaque* clear glass bottle and stopper, 4" [10.2 cm], long slender form with gem-like stopper, gold label, unopened, in its box and outer box; *Ecusson* glass bottle and frosted glass stopper, 3.4" [8.6 cm], full and sealed, gold labels on front and neck, in its box. Two items. Est. $100.00-$150.00.

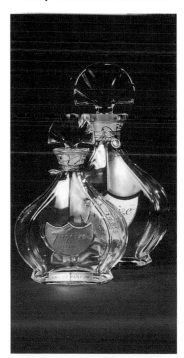

Lot #217. Corday *Trapèze* pair of identical shape glass bottles, 6.7" [17 cm] and 5.1" [13 cm], graceful curvilinear form on a pedestal base, fan stopper, empty, silver label on front of each which shows the "T" swinging from a trapeze. Two items. Est. $125.00-$175.00.

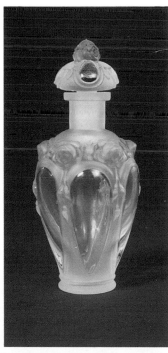

Lot #218. Coryse *Rose d'Ispahan* clear and frosted glass bottle and stopper, 5" [12.7 cm], the urn shape bottle molded with roses and clear oval windows, stopper of conforming design, traces of red patina, empty. Est. $300.00-$400.00.

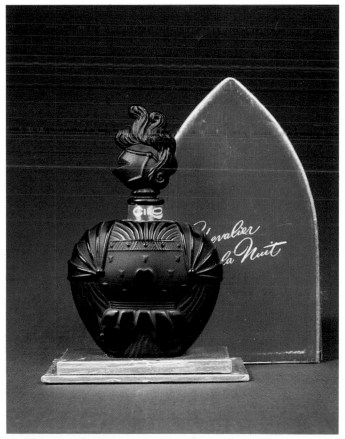

Lot #219. Ciro *Le Chevalier de la Nuit* ['Knight of the Night'] frosted black glass bottle and stopper formed as a stylized knight, 4.6" [11.7 cm], empty, pink label around neck, bottom marked dummy, in its pink and rose box whose shape is that of a knight's shield inverted. Est. $500.00-$600.00.

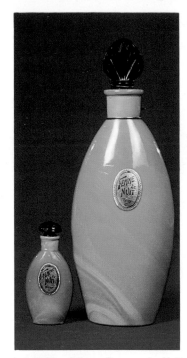

Lot #220. D'biny *Femme de Nuit* ['Woman of the Night', a French euphemism] green glass bottle and black glass stopper, 7" [17.8 cm], the opaque glass beautifully textured with wavy lines, empty, gold label on front; similar miniature bottle, 2.4" [6.2 cm], slightly different stopper, empty, gold label. Two items. Est. $300.00-$400.00.

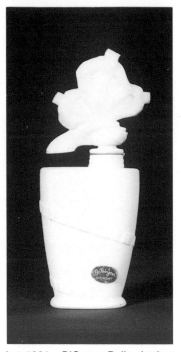

Lot #221. D'Orsay *Belle de Jour* white satin glass bottle and stopper, 5.5" [14 cm], the base entwined with molded ribbon, the stopper as a hand holding bows, empty, with its label near base. Est. $400.00-$500.00.

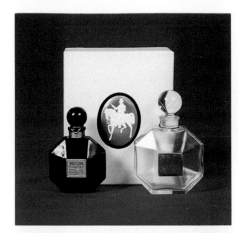

Lot #222. D'Orsay *Le Dandy* black glass bottle and stopper, 2.6" [6.6 cm], of octagonal pillow form with ball stopper, full and sealed, gold label, in its box; *Comtesse d'Orsay* clear glass bottle and stopper, 3" [7.6 cm], worn label, empty. Two items. Est. $150.00-$250.00.

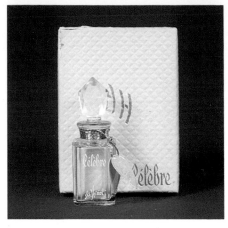

Lot #223. De Heriot *Célèbre* clear glass bottle and faceted ball stopper, 3.4" [8.6 cm], the stopper highly faceted, names in white enamel on front, gift tag "Forever in My Heart" around neck, empty, in its original box. Est. $100.00-$125.00.

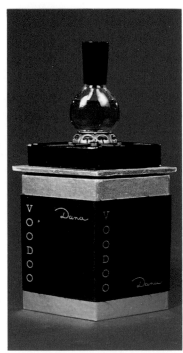

Lot #224. Dana *Voodoo* clear glass bottle with black cap mounted on a metal base, 2.7" [6.8 cm], with perfume, in a diamond shaped box of black and gold with red satin. This fragrance, probably unsuccessful in its time, dates from the early 1950's. Est. $100.00-$125.00.

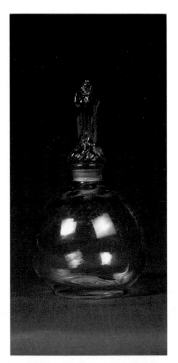

Lot #225. De Raymond *Deviltry* pink glass bottle and red glass stopper, 5" [12.7 cm], the bottle basically of spherical shape, the stopper as a standing figure of Mephistopheles, label on base, empty. Est. $600.00-$700.00.

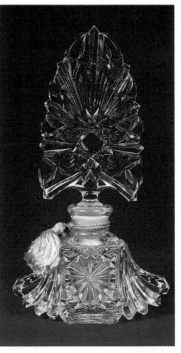

Lot #226. Deleith *Ellen's Secret* an American pressed glass perfume bottle and stopper, 6.9" [17.5 cm], molded so as to mimic the facets of cut glass, empty, tassels around neck, labels on neck, bottom label of Irving Rice; this was undoubtedly a wartime production when Czech glass could no longer be imported. Est. $75.00-$150.00.

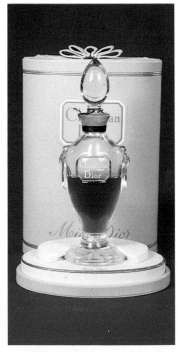

Lot #227. Christian Dior *Miss Dior* clear glass bottle and stopper, 4.5" [11.4 cm], the bottle shaped as an urn with two molded rings on either side, some perfume, name in white enamel on front, in its gray box decorated with ribbon. Est. $150.00-$250.00.

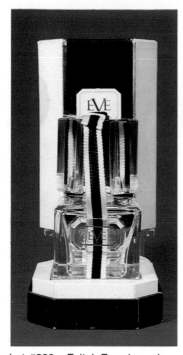

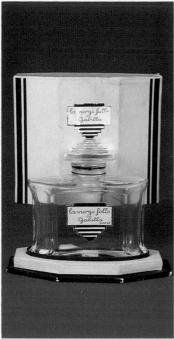

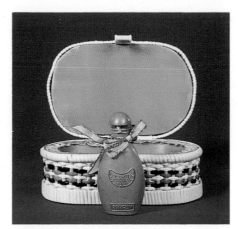

Lot #230. Duvelle *Le Gui* ['Mistletoe'] clear glass bottle and stopper, 3.2" [8.1 cm], the bottle entirely enameled in violet, gold labels on bottle and neck with ribbon bow, full and sealed, in its green and white wicker basket also marked Duvelle. Est. $100.00-$150.00.

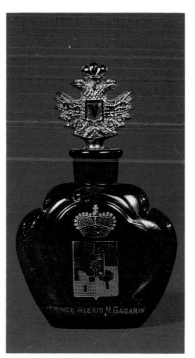

Lot #231. Fragonard *Moment Volé* ['Stolen Moment'] clear glass bottle and stopper, 3.5" [8.9 cm], the rectangular bottle decorated with geometric motifs, pink label on stopper, full and sealed, in its white and pink box; larger bottle of same design with gold cap, 5" [12.7 cm], full, in a pink box [price tag blemish on top of box]. Two items. Est. $125.00-$175.00.

Lot #228. Evital *Eve* clear glass bottle and stopper of very unusual and intricate design, 3.5" [8.8 cm], the massive stopper shaped like a cross, glass medallion on front of bottle with its name under which a ribbon passes to unite the bottle and stopper, empty, in its box. Est. $100.00-$150.00.

Lot #229. Gabilla *La Vierge Folle* ['The Crazy Virgin'] clear glass bottle and stopper, 3.2" [8.1 cm], the bottle of oval shape, stopper with step motif, label on front, empty, in its blue and pink box with conforming label on front. Est. $350.00-$450.00.

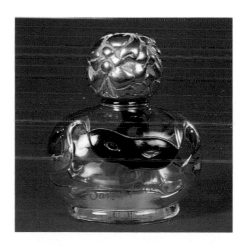

Lot #232. Dorothy Gray *Savoir Faire* clear glass bottle and gold metallic cap, 3.9" (9.9 cm), a highly original design of masks enameled in black and gold, cap molded as bows overlapping each other, empty, name enameled in front in gold, silver label on bottom. Est. $350.00-$450.00.

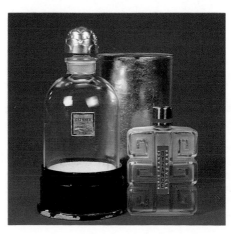

Lot #233. Grenoville *Byzance* frosted glass bottle, inner glass stopper and brass overcap, 3.5" [8.9 cm], the bottle molded with a Greek key motif, half-full and sealed, red label on front; glass bottle and stopper, 5.8" [14.7 cm], bottle of beehive shape, stopper with fishscale motif and covered in gold enamel, label on front, empty, in its gold box. Two items. Est. $150.00-$200.00.

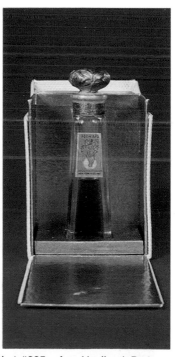

Lot #234. Prince Alexis N. Gagarin blue glass bottle and stopper, 3.7" [9.4 cm], the bottle with a gold enamel design of a crown and coat of arms, the stopper molded as the Russian Imperial double eagle and enameled in gold, empty. Est. $150.00-$250.00.

Lot #235. Ann Haviland *Perhaps* clear glass bottle and stopper, 3.9" [10 cm], the bottle of slender rectangular shape, stopper molded with flowers and completely covered in gold enamel, full and sealed, gold label with a hand holding flowers, in its drop-front box. Est. $150.00-$200.00.

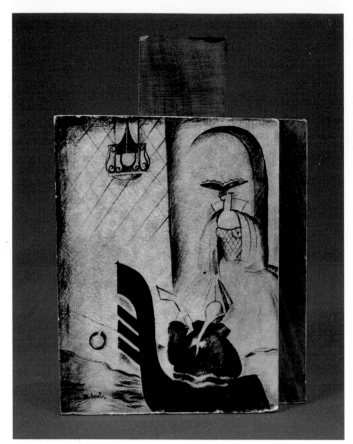

Lot #236. Grenoville *Casanova* rare glass bottle and stopper with wood overcap, 4" [10.2 cm], the bottle entirely encased in a wood base [fruitwood or walnut] upon which is laminated a beautiful graphic showing Casanova in a gondola singing to a Venetian lady, artwork signed M. Bovis; label laminated on side, empty. Est. $400.00-$500.00.

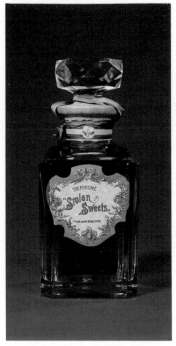

Lot #237. Hilberts *Stolen Sweets* clear glass bottle and stopper of very large size, 7" [17.8 cm], shaped as a liquor decanter and almost as big, faceted gem-like stopper, full and sealed, pretty label on front and on side, possibly a store display item; made by A. J. Hilbert Co., Milwaukee. Est. $125.00-$200.00.

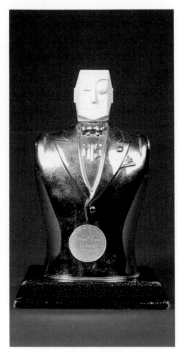

Lot #238. House for Men *HIS* clear glass bottle and white plastic stopper molded as a man in tuxedo with square, stylized face, 6.25" [15.9 cm], full, the bottle entirely covered in gold enamel, gold label on front, mounted on a cardboard base. Cf. Lefkowith, p. 177, #204. Est. $150.00-$250.00.

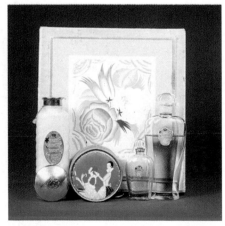

Lot #239. Richard Hudnut *Three Flowers* gift set of five items, perfume 3.7" [9.4 cm] [evaporated], toilet water 6.2" [15.8 cm], talc, face powder, and compact, all unused except for compact, in a deluxe gift box of silver and peach. Est. $150.00-$250.00.

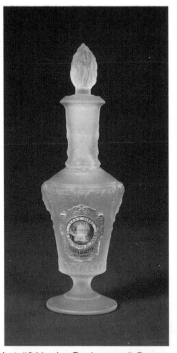

Lot #241. La Duchessa di Parma *Vera Violetta* frosted glass bottle and stopper, 5.2" [13.2 cm], shaped interestingly as a vase or urn with flame stopper, classical heads molded on either side, empty, pretty gold and green label with portrait presumably of the Duchess. Est. $150.00-$250.00.

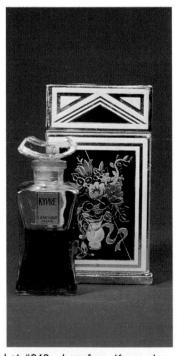

Lot #242. Lancôme *Kypre* clear glass bottle and stopper, 3.2" [8 cm], bottle basically rectangular but with indented sides, stopper an arc, some perfume, gold label, in its highly decorative gold foil box. Est. $150.00-$200.00.

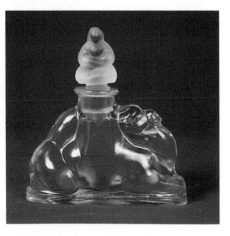

Lot #240. Jovoy *Severem* clear glass bottle and frosted glass stopper in the form of a camel and rider, 3.6" [9.1 cm], some perfume, [label lacking], bottom molded © *Lordonnais 1922 France*. Est. $400.00-$500.00.

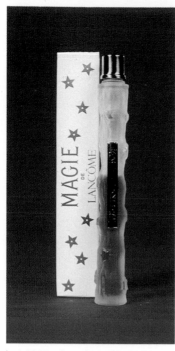

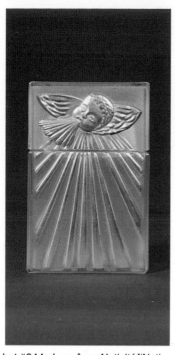

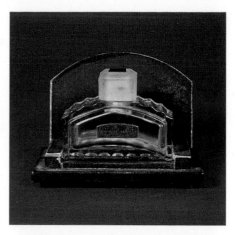

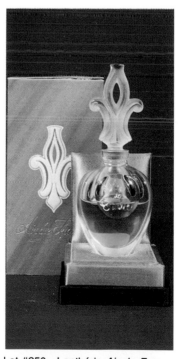

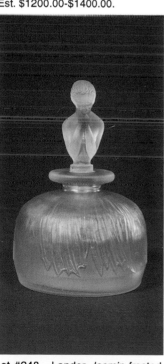

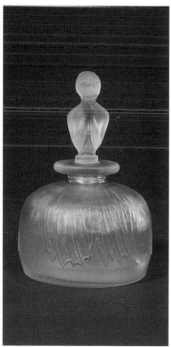

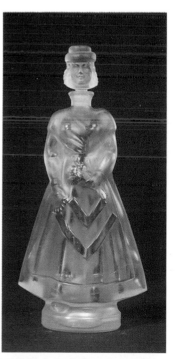

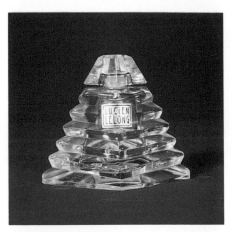

Lot #251. Lucien Lelong *Opening Night* clear glass bottle and stopper, 2.7" [6.9 cm], the bottle of pyramid shape with steps, empty, with its silver Lucien Lelong label on front, Lelong logo molded into base, acid mark France. Est. $350.00-$450.00.

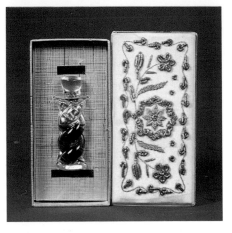

Lot #252. Lucien Lelong *Sirôcco* clear glass bottle and ground glass stopper, 7.8" [19 cm], the column shape of interlocking swirls of glass, with perfume and sealed, tiny gold label at base, in a very unusual gold box with gold beaded decoration on top. Est. $350.00-$450.00.

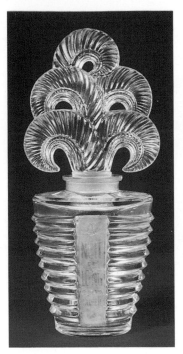

Lot #253. Lubin *Nuit de Longchamps* clear glass bottle and stopper, 6" [15.2 cm], bottle molded with concentric rings, label on front [worn], elaborate stopper molded as plumes or stylized feathers, empty, signed Lubin on base. Est. $125.00-$175.00.

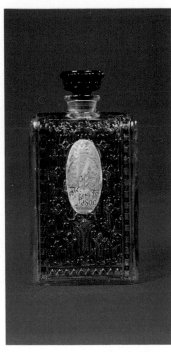

Lot #254. Myrurgia *Flor de Blason* unusual clear glass bottle and black glass crown stopper, 3.4" [8.6 cm], with an arabesque design molded on both sides of the bottle, enameled in the recesses in light blue, gold label marked Myrurgia Barcelona, empty. Est. $200.00-$300.00.

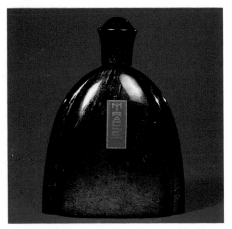

Lot #255. Lenthéric *Miracle* very large size black glass bottle and stopper with black composition overcap, 5.8" [14.7 cm], a unique design made by putting gold inclusions in the glass, empty, red label on front. Est. $400.00-$500.00.

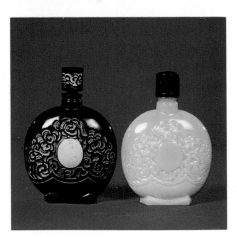

Lot #256. Lionceau *Le Fleuve Noir* ['Black River'] black glass bottle and stopper, 3.1" [7.9 cm], oval shape with an abstract motif of swirls molded around the bottle, blue patina, empty, silver label [faint], signed Lionceau; similar bottle of green glass with black screw-on cap, empty, label lacking, signed Lionceau. Two items. Est. $400.00-$500.00.

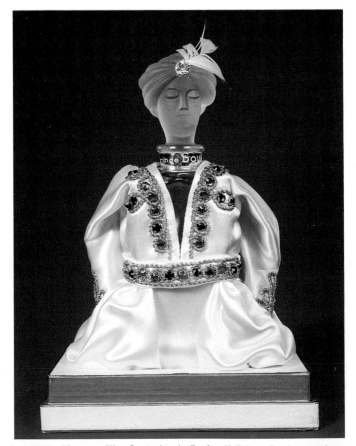

Lot #257. Marquay ["Le Couturier du Parfum"] *Prince Douka* very large size clear glass bottle and frosted glass stopper, 6.2" [15.7 cm], designed in the shape of a swami, cream satin cape decorated elaborately with rhinestones; clear rhinestone in center of turban, empty, in its box bottom. Est. $450.00-$550.00.

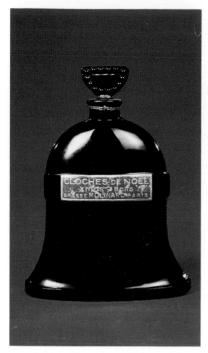

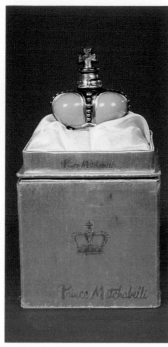

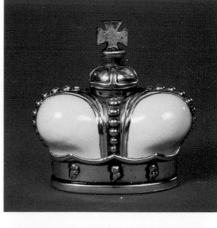

Lot #260. Matchabelli *Belovèd* large size opaque green glass bottle and clear glass stopper, 3.8" [9.7 cm], the green glass of the crown shape also enameled in gold [some wear to gold but overall good condition], empty, gold label on base. Est. $350.00-$450.00.

Lot #258. Molinard *Les Cloches de Noël - Xmas Bells* black glass bottle and stopper, 4.2" [10.7 cm], shaped as the silhouette of a bell, red and silver metallic label, full and sealed. Est. $200.00-$300.00.

Lot #259. Matchabelli *Belovèd* glass bottle and stopper in the crown shape, 2.2" [5.5 cm], enameled in sky blue and gold, label on bottom, empty, in its rectangular box. Est. $125.00-$200.00.

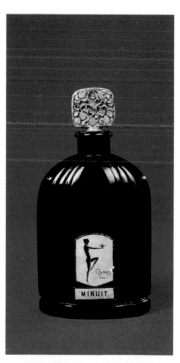

Lot #261. Melba [unidentified fragrance] clear and frosted glass bottle and stopper, 4.9" [12.5 cm], the stopper molded with flowers and leaves, the bottle front with a panel depicting a nude woman and her lover, 'Melba' a part of the design, back of bottle molded Melba, empty. Est. $150.00-$250.00.

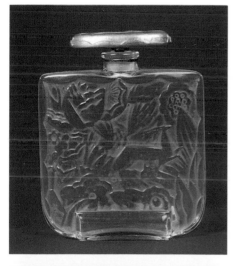

Lot #262. Lubin *Monjoly* clear glass bottle and stopper, 3.9" [10 cm], of flat flask shape, the entire front surface molded with an Art Deco tableau of a gazelle amid fantastic plants, stopper covered in gold enamel, empty, label lacking, bottom signed Lubin. Est. $250.00-$350.00.

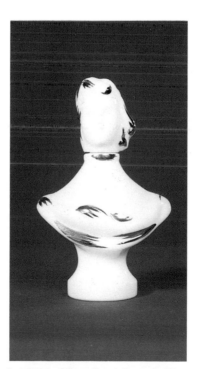

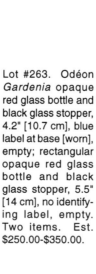

Lot #263. Odéon *Gardenia* opaque red glass bottle and black glass stopper, 4.2" [10.7 cm], blue label at base [worn], empty; rectangular opaque red glass bottle and black glass stopper, 5.5" [14 cm], no identifying label, empty. Two items. Est. $250.00-$350.00.

Lot #264. Gilbert Orcel *Coup de Chapeau* ['Tip of the Hat'] white glass bottle, inner stopper and overcap, 5" [12.5 cm], molded as the bust of a woman, highlights enameled in gold, empty, bottom molded Orcel Made in France. Est. $175.00-$250.00.

Lot #265. Ramey *Minuit* ['Midnight'] black glass bottle and stopper, 4.3" [11 cm], label shows a nude woman holding a perfume burner, stopper molded with berries and covered in gold enamel, traces of perfume. Est. $250.00-$350.00.

Lot #266. Prince de Chany *Mystery Gardenia* clear glass bottle, inner stopper, and overcap, 2.6" [6.6 cm], the bottle molded with grooved lines in an abstract geometric pattern and patinated gray in the recesses, silver label, empty; *Lost Orchid* clear glass bottle and crown-form stopper, 4.2" [10.7 cm], silver label also with crown, empty. Two items. Est. $250.00-$350.00.

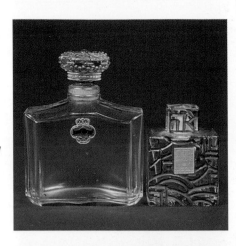

Lot #267. Rigaud *Marthe Chenal* clear glass bottle and black glass stopper, 3.9" [10 cm], full and sealed, gold label on bottle and on box, in its pink and gold box; *Un Air Embaumé* clear and frosted glass bottle and stopper, 2.6" [6.6 cm], molded design of women on sides of bottle, peach patination overall, gold label on front, empty, in its bright peach box and outer box. Two items. Est. $275.00-$400.00.

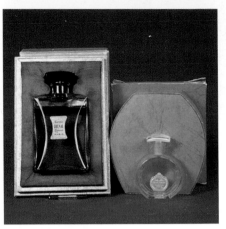

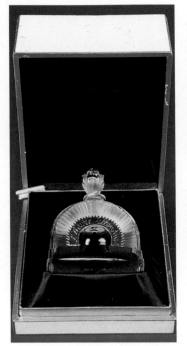

Lot #268. Jean Patou *L'Heure Attendue* ['The Awaited Hour'] clear and frosted glass bottle and stopper, 2.8" [7.1 cm], the bottle molded as the rising sun, floriform stopper, full and sealed, gold label on front, Patou label on back, signed, in a beautiful écru box with deep blue satin lining. This perfume is historically important as it commemorates the liberation of France. Est. $250.00-$350.00.

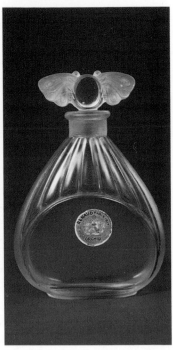

Lot #269. Renaud *Orchid* fine quality clear and frosted glass bottle and stopper, 4.3" [11 cm], the bottle shaped like a butterfly wing, the stopper molded as two butterflies, empty, gold label, traces of violet patina. Est. $400.00-$500.00.

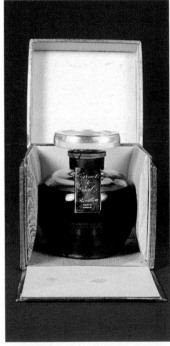

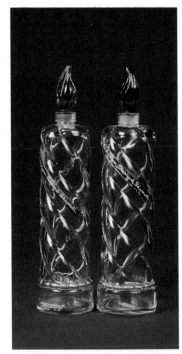

Lot #272. Schiaparelli *Salut* clear glass bottle and stopper, 2.1" [5.3 cm], full and sealed, blue label on front and "S" logo enameled onto top of stopper, in a molded white lily holder signed Schiaparelli. Est. $100.00-$150.00.

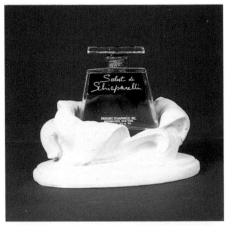

Lot #270. Revillon *Carnet de Bal* large size clear glass bottle and stopper, 3.5" [9 cm], the bottle and stopper shaped as a brandy snifter inverted, Revillon logo intaglio molded into top of stopper, with perfume, gold metal 'dance card' label, in its box which has interior perfume stains. Est. $125.00-$175.00.

Lot #271. Schiaparelli *Sleeping* pair of identical clear glass bottles with reddish amber glass stoppers, 7.6" [19.3 cm], molded in the shape of a candle with swirls, empty, gold label following the curve of the glass, gold enamel beads at base, both signed Schiaparelli in the mold. Two items. Est. $150.00-$250.00.

Lot #273. Schiaparelli *Shocking* pair of clear glass bottles and stoppers in the form of a dress dummy, each in its glass dome which is 4.7" [12 cm], tape measure labels [stained], both empty, one with glass flowers and one with plastic ones. Two items. Est. $200.00-$300.00.

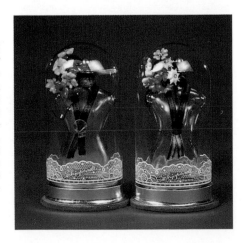

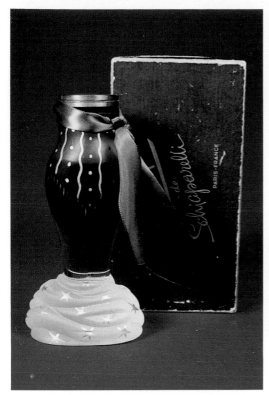

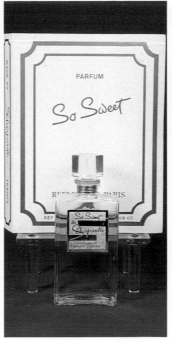

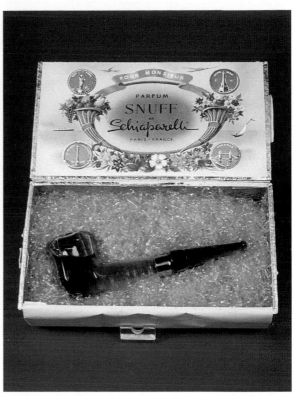

Lot #274. Schiaparelli *Zut* ['Damn!!'] glass bottle and stopper in the shape of a woman's torso from the waist downward, 4.9" [12.4 cm], panties and base frosted, detail enameled in gold, gold enameled stopper with name in black, waist tied with green ribbon, with perfume, in its seldom seen green box lined with violet silk. Est. $500.00-$650.00.

Lot #275. Schiaparelli *So Sweet* clear glass bottle and stopper, 3.7" [9.4 cm], rectangular form with cube stopper, gold label on front, unopened, in its gold book-form box. This is a very seldom seen Schiaparelli fragrance, and unusual in that it is devoid of pink. Est. $75.00-$150.00.

Lot #276. Schiaparelli *Snuff* clear glass bottle and amber glass stopper in the form of a pipe, 5.4" long [13.7 cm], full and sealed, the stopper molded Schiaparelli, decal label on bowl of pipe, in its original box designed as if for cigars. Est. $250.00-$350.00.

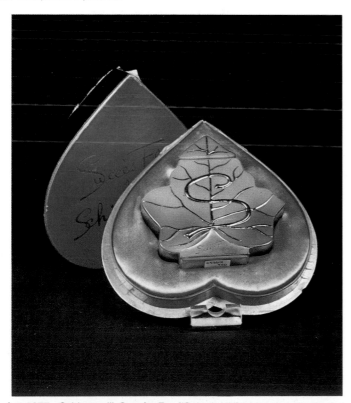

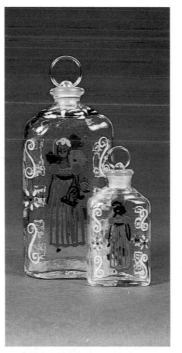

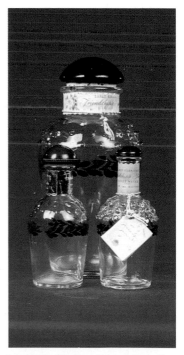

Lot #277. Schiaparelli *Succès Fou* ['Smash Hit'] white glass bottle and screw-on cap in the shape of a fig leaf, 3" [7.6 cm], empty, the entire bottle enameled in green and gold, bottom molded Schiaparelli, in its seldom seen pink and green box lined with pink satin. Est. $800.00-$1000.00.

Lot #278. Shulton *Early American* pair of clear glass bottles and stoppers, 5" [12.7 cm] and 2.9" [7.4 cm], the glass made with an antique, hand-blown quality, both colorfully decorated with a maiden carrying flowers in a basket, empty, no labels; the larger size bottle is quite difficult to find. Est. $150.00-$250.00.

Lot #279. Shulton *Friendship's Garden* ensemble of three bottles, one 7" [17.8 cm] and two 4.1" [10.4 cm], all empty, labels around necks, glass made by the Wheaton Glass Co. Three items. Est. $75.00-$150.00.

Lot #280. Seely [Detroit] *Purple Lilac* clear glass bottle and stopper, 4.2" [10.7 cm], empty, beautiful label on front, US tax stamp on the reverse dated 1898, in its box [worn]; Vallant *Carnation* clear glass bottle and glass cork-tipped stopper, 5.5" [14 cm], empty, pretty label, in a beautiful box decorated with oriental poppies. Two items. Est. $150.00-$200.00.

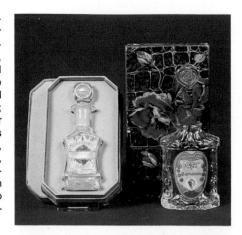

Lot #281. Mira Talka turquoise glass bottle and turquoise lucite stopper, 3.5" [8.9 cm], the bottle mounted with a gold breastplate and enameled with necklaces meant to resemble Egyptian jewelry, full, in its turquoise box with Egyptian lotus motifs. Est. $100.00-$150.00.

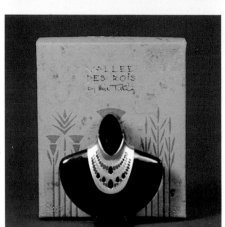

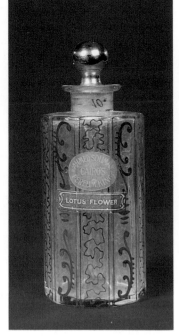

Lot #282. Ahmed Soliman *Lotus Flower* clear glass bottle and stopper, 5" [12.7 cm], the column form of the bottle molded with ten panels, each enameled with an abstract gold design, ball stopper with long dauber enameled in gold, empty, labels on front, the glass possibly of Bohemian manufacture. Est. $350.00-$450.00.

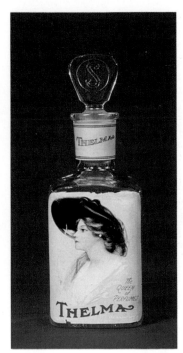

Lot #283. Stearns [Detroit, Michigan] *Thelma* 'The Queen of Perfumes' clear glass bottle and stopper, 7" [17.8 cm], the bottle rectangular with long neck, S impressed into stopper, bottom of bottle molded Stearns etc., front label with a beautiful early 20th century graphic of a woman in large black hat [minor fraying of label edges], empty. Est. $50.00-$85.00.

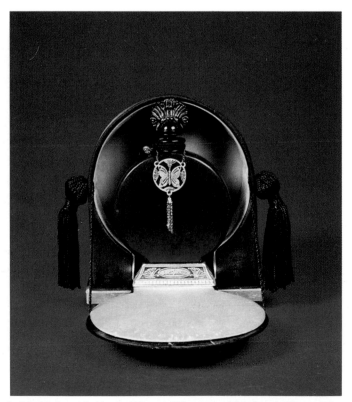

Lot #284. Lucretia Vanderbilt cased blue over white glass bottle and blue glass stopper, 4.7" [12 cm], the bottle mounted on a silver metal base, stopper with long dauber, butterfly medallion around the neck, empty, in its beautiful drop-front box of blue and cream satin [new tassels] box [with some wear] on four metal feet. Est. $1250.00-$1500.00.

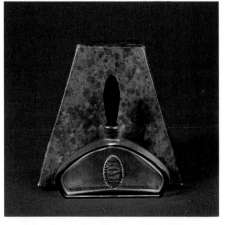

Lot #285. Varquer *Azatecs Negros* clear and frosted crystal bottle and black glass stopper, 3.4" [8.6 cm], empty, faceted stopper, gold label on front also marked Mazatlan, possibly of Bohemian manufacture, in an interesting blue and red box. Est. $350.00-$450.00.

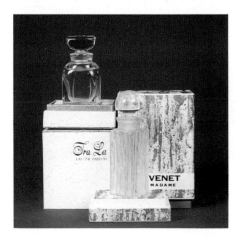

Lot #286. Philippe Venet *Madame* frosted glass bottle with clear glass ball stopper with plastic tip, 4.3" [10.9 cm], bottle molded with vines, empty, in its box; Colonial Dames *Tra La* clear glass bottle and stopper, 3.1" [7.9 cm], gold label on base, bottom molded France, with perfume, in its cream and gold box. Two items. Est. $50.00-$100.00.

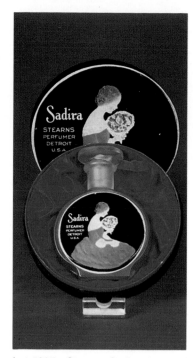

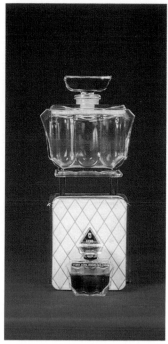

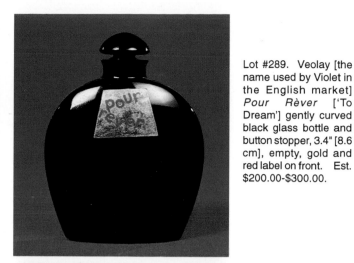

Lot #287. Stearns *Sadira* clear and frosted glass bottle and stopper, 3.3" [8.4 cm], the bottle of round flat shape, stopper with molded flowers, front of bottle covered entirely with a beautiful label showing a seated lady with a bouquet of flowers, empty, in its black box lined with red satin and bearing the same graphic design. Est. $125.00-$175.00.

Lot #288. Vigny *Echo Troublant* clear glass bottle and stopper, 2.4" [6 cm], bottle in a coat of arms shape, Vigny logo molded into stopper, full and sealed, thin gold label, in its box; identical large size cologne bottle, 4.8" [12.2 cm], empty, with label [faded]. Two items. Est. $125.00-$200.00.

Lot #289. Veolay [the name used by Violet in the English market] *Pour Rêver* ['To Dream'] gently curved black glass bottle and button stopper, 3.4" [8.6 cm], empty, gold and red label on front. Est. $200.00-$300.00.

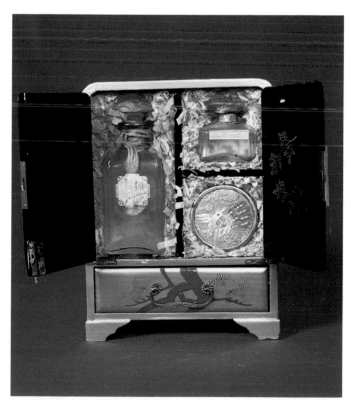

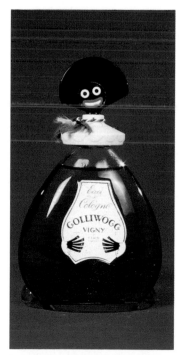

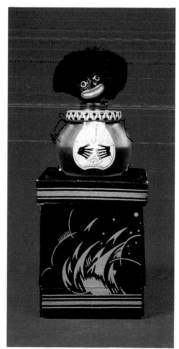

Lot #290. Vantine's *Van San* and *Mikado* clear glass bottles with frosted glass stoppers, 2" [5.1 cm], the bottle having a pagoda-like appearance, empty, gold labels on front, in a Japanese lacquerware box with blue velvet lining also bearing a Vantine's gold label and signed on bottom. Est. $175.00-$250.00.

Lot #291. Vantine's *Chypre* set: clear glass bottle and frosted cork-tipped stopper, 4.7" [11.9 cm], empty, silver label; smaller bottle, 2" [5.1 cm], empty, gold label; unused silver metal compact with inset brocade; all in a deluxe lacquerware jewelry chest, with drawer, lock, and key. Rare to find so complete and in this condition. Est. $400.00-$500.00.

Lot #292. Vigny *Golliwogg Eau de Cologne* glass bottle and plastic cap, 6.5" [16.5 cm], a 1940's interpretation of the Golliwogg design [actually much less often seen than its older counterpart], full, label on front. Est. $225.00-$300.00.

Lot #293. Vigny *Le Golliwogg* beautiful medium size frosted glass bottle and black glass stopper, 3.4" [8.5 cm] to top of hair, molded as a Golliwogg, some perfume, crisp label on front, in its box lined in brilliant pink silk. Excellent condition in this larger size. Est. $500.00-$600.00.

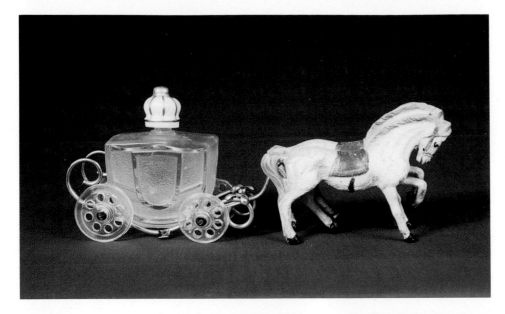

Lot #294. Jean Welle charming clear and frosted glass bottle and white screw-on cap, 3.4" [8.6 cm], bottle molded as a carriage, empty, base signed Jean Welle, fitted into a set of wheels and drawn by two composition horses. A superb novelty presentation. Est. $250.00-$400.00.

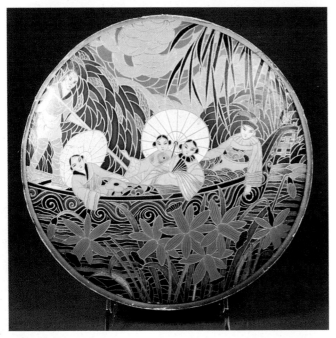

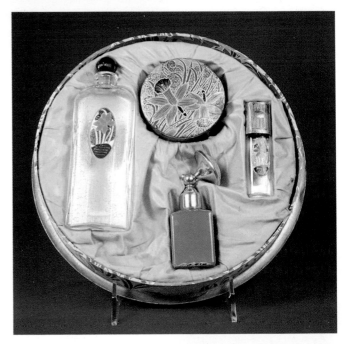

Lot #295. Vivadoux *Narcisse de Chine* deluxe boxed set of four items: Eau de Toilette clear glass ribbed bottle with amber ball stopper, 6" [15.2 cm], ornate powder box [empty], DeVilbiss perfume atomizer of square shape enameled in blue, perfume bottle with glass stopper and brass overcap, 3.2" [8.1 cm], in a beautifully decorated box showing Chinese ladies in a boat [small piece of paper torn away on side of box]. Est. $650.00-$750.00.

Lot #296. Yardley *Flair* clear glass bottle and frosted glass stopper, 1.6" [4.1 cm], of highly unusual free-form shape with three sides, with perfume, gold label on stopper, in a box decorated continuously with scarf dancers. Est. $100.00-$150.00.

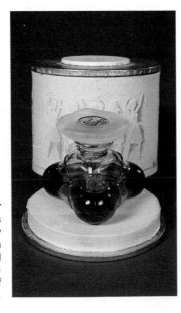

FRENCH ART GLASS MASTERS:

M. DÉPINOIX
L. GAILLARD
A. JOLLIVET
R. LALIQUE
J. VIARD, ET ALIA

Lot #297. Violet *Ambre Royal* clear glass bottle and black glass stopper, 2.5" [6.4 cm], the bottle molded with inset panels stained brown, some perfume [stopper frozen], Lucien Gaillard logo molded on base. Est. $200.00-$300.00.

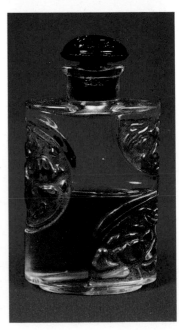

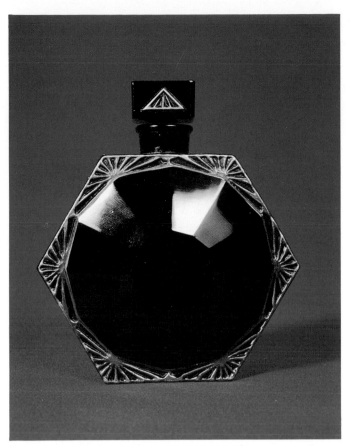

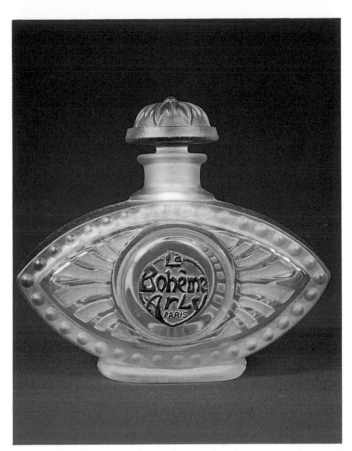

Lot #298. Unidentified perfumer and fragrance, black glass bottle and stopper, 4" [10.2 cm], the bottle of clockform shape within a hexagon, the ray motif of the bottle continued around edge and on stopper, recesses enameled in silver, acid-etched Made in France. Est. $700.00-$850.00.

Lot #299. Arly *La Bohème* Eau de Toilette clear and frosted glass bottle and stopper, 4" [10.2 cm], the bottle shaped as an eye with an abstract design on both sides and with a clear round window at center, empty, labels front and back, by M. Dépinoix, unsigned. Est. $300.00-$450.00.

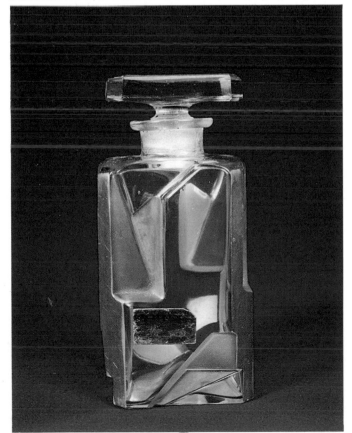

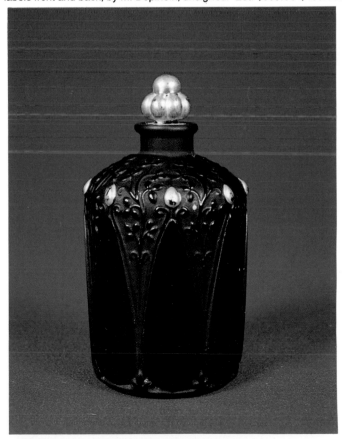

Lot #300. De Seghers *Pinx* clear and frosted glass bottle, 3.9" [10 cm], molded on all sides with abstract geometric motifs in the cubist style, some facets frosted or enameled in gold, labels front and back [worn and faint], bottom signed A. Jollivet in acid. Est. $500.00-$600.00.

Lot #301. Atkinsons [unidentified fragrance] fine quality black glass bottle and stopper, 3" [7.6 cm], the bottle with polished facets of teardrop shape on eight sides and decorated with molded berries and vines, part of the design enameled in gold, partial label, empty. Est. $600.00-$750.00.

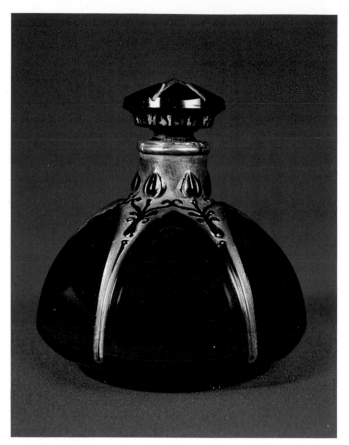

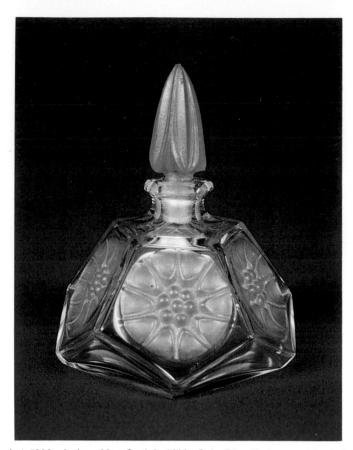

Lot #302. Godet *Nuit d'Amour* cobalt blue glass bottle and stopper, 3" [7.6 cm], the bottle of hexagonal form with six polished windows, stopper with conforming design, recesses enameled in silver, empty, no label, bottom acid-etched France in circle. Est. $700.00-$850.00.

Lot #303. Isabey *Mon Seul Ami* ['My Only Friend'] clear and frosted glass bottle, 3.4" [8.6 cm], designed with five pentagonal windows inset with a flower, with the stopper molded with leaves, rich amber patina, bottle by Bobin Frères, possibly a J. Viard design. Est. $600.00-$700.00.

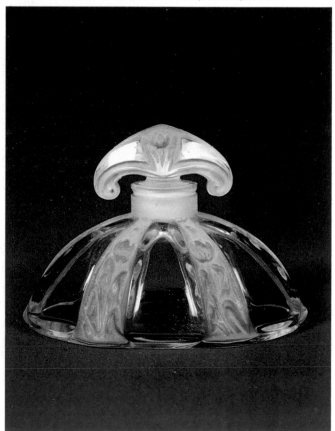

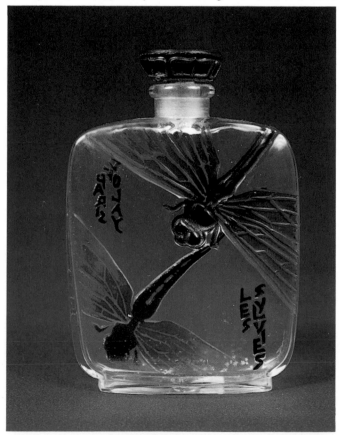

Lot #304. Unidentified perfumer and fragrance, clear and frosted glass bottle and stopper, 2.3" [5.8 cm], the bottle beautifully designed with panels of flowers and clear glass windows, amber patina, empty, acid marked Made in France in circle, unsigned. Est. $700.00-$850.00.

Lot #305. Veolay [=Violet] *Les Sylvies* clear glass bottle and stopper of flask shape, 3.6" [9.1 cm], a design of dragonflies molded onto the front and back, blue and black patina, names on front and on reverse, signed with LG logo [Lucien Gaillard], empty. Est. $1250.00-$1750.00.

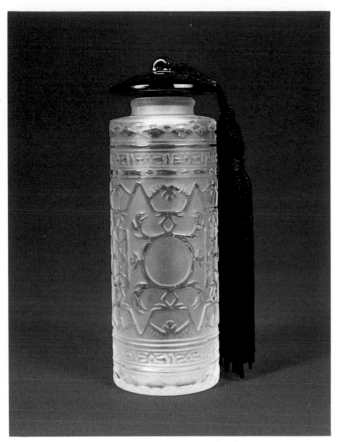

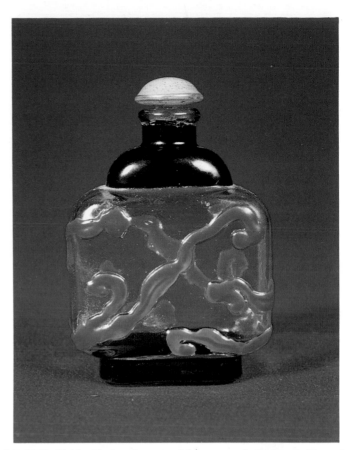

Lot #306. Rosine *1925* clear and frosted glass bottle and red glass stopper, 4.8" [12.2 cm], the bottle of column shape decorated with molded oriental motifs, coolie-hat stopper with black tassel, empty, label lacking, by M. Dépinoix, unsigned. Est. $700.00-$850.00.

Lot #307. Unidentified perfumer and fragrance, clear glass bottle and stopper, 2.7" [6.9 cm], designed as an oriental snuff bottle, molded scrolls enameled in bright coral, base and neck in black, and stopper in green, empty, bottom molded J. Viard. Est. $1000.00-$1200.00.

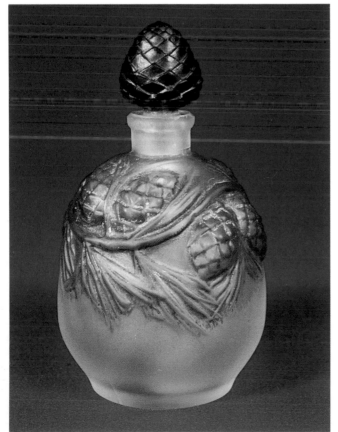

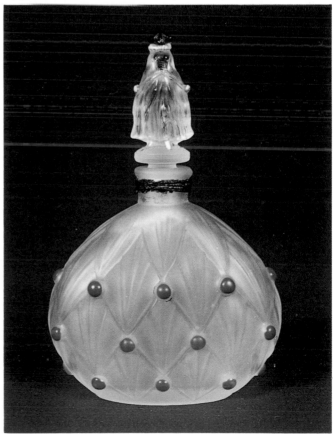

Lot #308. Odéon *Pour Amour* ['For Love'] frosted glass bottle and stopper, 3.6" [9.1 cm], the bottle molded with pine branches and pine cones, the stopper designed as a single pine cone, empty, rich grayish green patina, label on bottom, possibly by J. Viard. Est. $800.00-$1000.00.

Lot #309. Favolys *Glyciane* frosted glass bottle and stopper, 3.5" [8.9 cm], the bottle molded with layers of leaves and blue enameled balls [small imperfections on lip], the stopper an elegant Venetian lady; empty, gold label, signed in the mold J. Viard. Est. $1750.00-$2000.00.

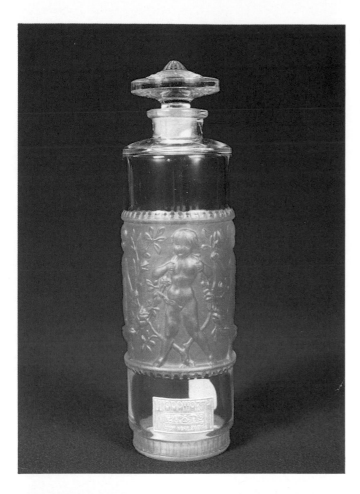

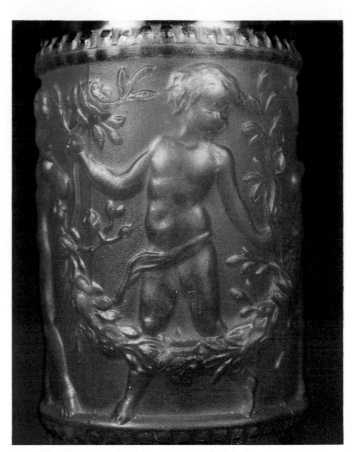

Lot #310. Woodworth *Tous Les Bouquets* ['All the Bouquets'], clear and frosted glass bottle of cylinder shape, 5" [12.7 cm], the bottle with a frieze of children amid garlands of flowers highlighted with rich brown patina, the stopper with a floral design, empty, label on bottom and gold label on front of bottle [both in pristine condition], bottom molded J. Viard; overall condition is superb. Cf. Lefkowith, p. 127, #107. Est. $1000.00-$1250.00.

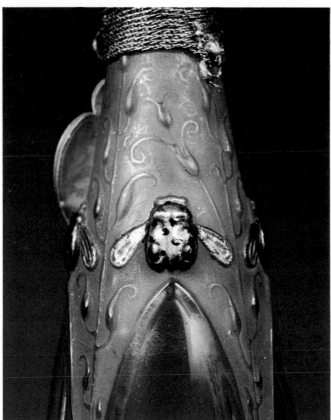

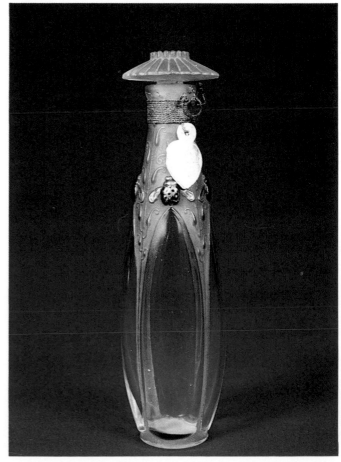

Lot #311. Caray *Parfum Caray* clear and frosted glass bottle and stopper, 6" [15.3 cm], the bottle of slender form with tall oval windows molded on four sides, upper portion of bottle with a design of leaves and beetles enameled realistically in iridescent green, empty, tag around neck, unsigned. Not seen in available reference works. Est. $2500.00-$3000.00.

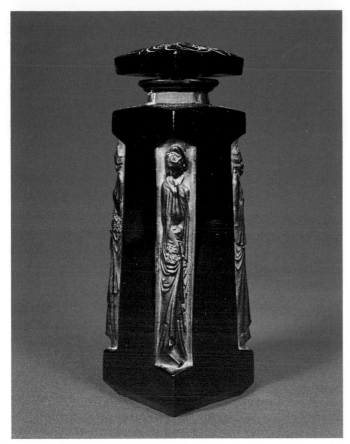

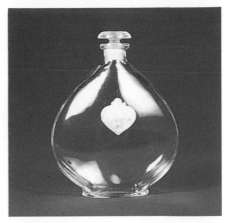

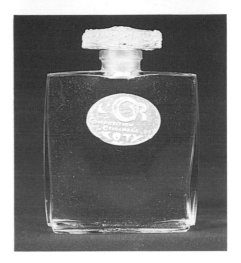

Lot #312. D'Orsay *Ambre d'Orsay* black glass bottle and stopper, 5.2" [13.2 cm], of tall rectangular form with classical maidens in the four corners and appearing as caryatids, stopper molded with flowers, edges molded *Lalique* and *Ambre d'Orsay*, empty. Utt #DO-1. Est. $2500.00-$3000.00.

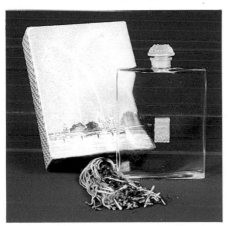

Lot #315. Coty *Paris* clear glass bottle and stopper, 3.5" [9 cm], a totally rectangular form which achieves elegance in simplicity, stopper molded with berries and leaves, empty, silver label on front, in a beautiful tasseled box [some stains] which spells the names in fireworks over the city of Paris, unsigned. Est. $300.00-$400.00.

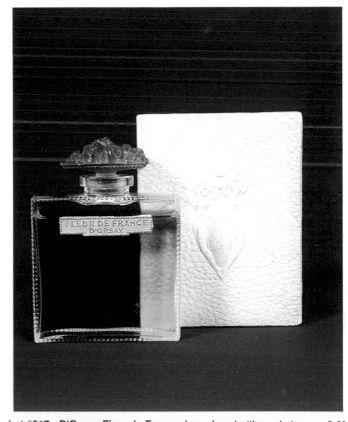

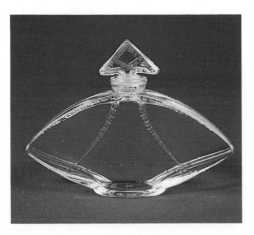

Lot #316. Houbigant *Ensemble* clear glass bottle and stopper, 2.3" [5.8 cm], of fan shape decorated with strands of flowers, empty [label lacking], molded R. Lalique on base. Utt #H-3. Est. $500.00-$650.00.

Lot #317. D'Orsay *Fleur de France* clear glass bottle and stopper, 3.3" [8.4 cm], the rectangular form outlined with a border of beads, the stopper molded as a bouquet of flowers, gold label, full of perfume, signed R. Lalique in the mold, in its cream colored box decorated with nudes. Utt #DO-8. Est. $1200.00-$1500.00.

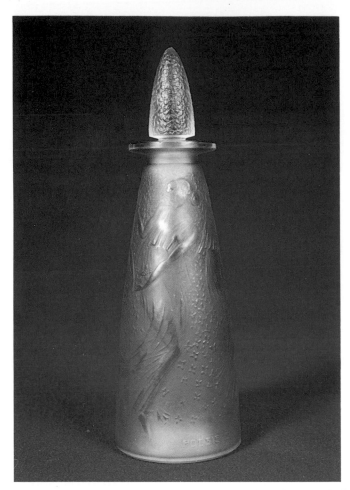

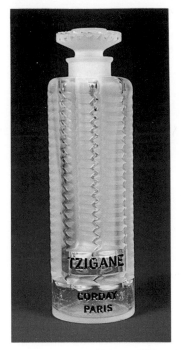

Lot #319. Corday *Tsigane* ['Gypsy'] very large size clear and frosted bottle and stopper, 6.9" [17.5 cm], indented zigzag design on a columnar form, names enameled in black near base, empty, molded signature R. Lalique. Utt #Cor-1. Est. $750.00-$1000.00.

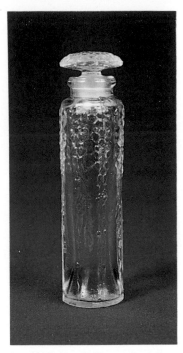

Lot #320. Forvil *Chypre* clear glass bottle and stopper of diminutive size, 3" [7.6 cm], of columnar shape molded with garlands of flowers cascading on all sides of the bottle, empty, bottom signed R. Lalique in the mold. Utt #F-7. Est. $300.00-$400.00.

Lot #318. D'Orsay *Poésie d'Orsay* frosted glass bottle and stopper, 5.9" [15 cm], both of cone shape, designed with classical maidens in diaphanous gowns dancing amid flowers, names molded near base, subtle blue patina, molded R. Lalique. Utt #DO-7. Est. $3000.00-$3500.00.

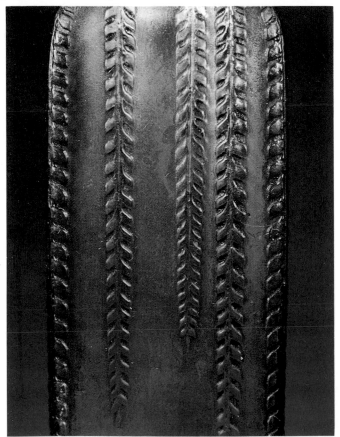

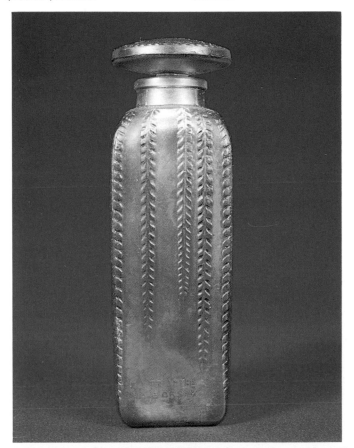

Lot #321. D'Orsay *Triomphe d'Orsay* frosted glass bottle and stopper, 4.7" [12 cm], the bottle a tall rectangular form with indented sides and molded with continuous wisteria vines, stopper with conforming design, rich purplish brown patina, names molded on side of bottle, signed R. Lalique in script. This model is identical to the Maison Lalique bottle called *Glycines* ['Wisteria.'], Utt #ML-513. Est. $3000.00-$4000.00.

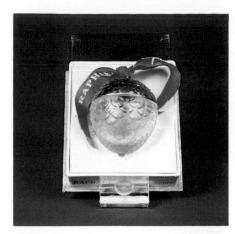

Lot #322. Raphael *Réplique* frosted glass bottle in the shape of an acorn with silver colored screw-on cap and red ribbon, 1.8" [4.6 cm], signed Lalique in black enamel under cap, in its original box with label on bottom. Est. $250.00-$350.00.

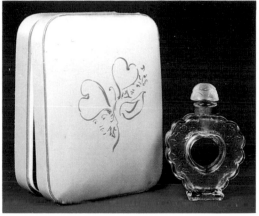

Lot #323. Nina Ricci *Coeur Joie* clear and frosted glass bottle in the form of a heart covered with small flowers, the stopper also with a butterfly, 4" [10 cm], some perfume, bottom etched Lalique France, in its earliest white satin box with white satin interior. Utt #NR-103. Est. $300.00-$400.00.

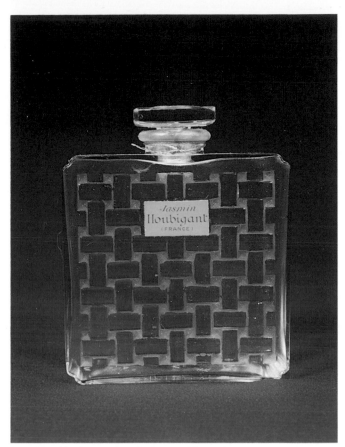

Lot #324. Houbigant *Jasmin* clear and frosted glass bottle and stopper, 3.2" [8.1 cm], of square shape with a basketweave motif on front and on stopper, empty, with its label, molded R. Lalique. Utt #H-6 [1922]. Est. $700.00-$850.00.

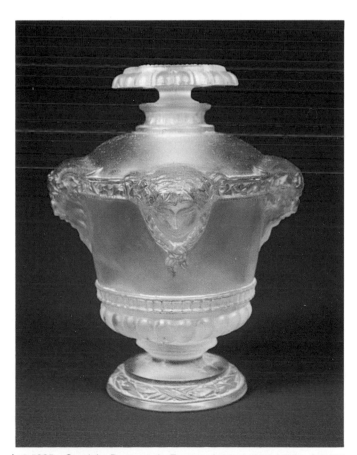

Lot #325. Guerlain *Bouquet de Faunes* frosted glass bottle, 4.3" [10 cm], molded as an urn with four sides decorated with faces of a woman or satyr on each corner, bottle molded Guerlain France, unsigned [as is normal for this bottle]. Utt #G-1. Est. $750.00-$900.00.

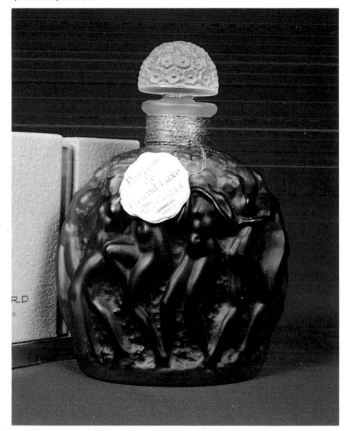

Lot #326. Molinard *Sketch* frosted glass bottle and stopper of beehive form, 4.5" [11.4 cm], the stopper molded with flowers, the bottle molded with nymphs, light brown patina, full and sealed, overall pristine condition, unsigned, box marked Flacon Lalique, in its deluxe presentation case and outer box. Utt #M-101. Est. $2000.00-$2500.00.

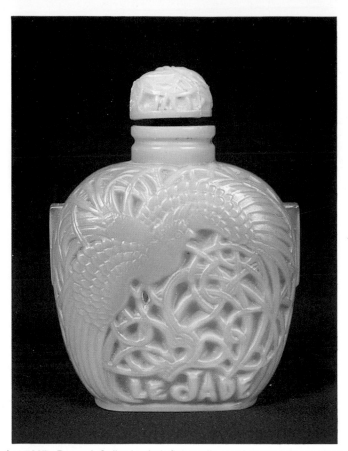

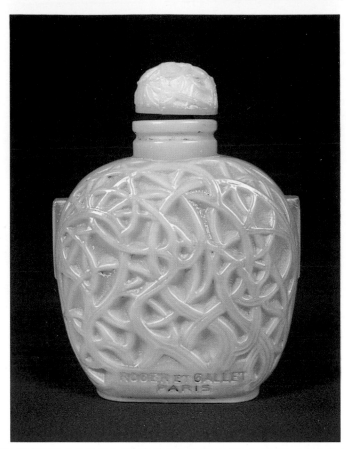

Lot #327. Roger & Gallet *Le Jade* fine quality semi-opaque green glass bottle and stopper, 3.2" [8.1 cm], the bottle designed to resemble an oriental snuff bottle, molded on one side with a bird with open wings amid vines and the words *Le Jade* as part of the design, and molded on the other side with intricate vines and the words Roger et Gallet Paris, signed R. L. on the base in the mold, empty. Utt #R&G-3. Est. $3000.00-$3500.00.

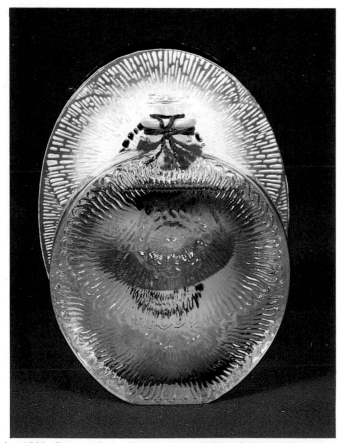

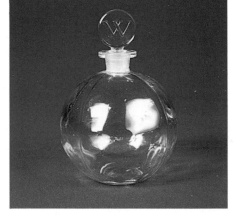

Lot #329. Worth *Dans la Nuit* clear glass bottle and stopper, 4.2" [10.7 cm], shaped as a sphere and decorated with molded stars, stopper with a molded W, empty, bottom signed R. Lalique in the mold. Utt #W-1. Est. $400.00-$500.00.

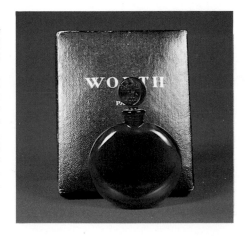

Lot #330. Worth *Dans La Nuit* ['In the Night'] blue glass bottle and stopper, 3.2" [8.1 cm], the bottle of flat round form with Worth molded on front, stopper molded with name and a crescent moon, empty, bottom molded R. Lalique, in its blue and cream satin box. Utt #W-2 Est. $500.00-$600.00.

Lot #328. Roger & Gallet *Pavots d'Argent* ['Silver Poppies'] clear glass bottle and stopper, 3.3" [8.4 cm], bottle molded in the form of two open poppies, stopper also molded as a flower, with perfume and still sealed, label on back, in its pink and silver box [small worn spot], signed faintly in the mold R. Lalique. Utt #R&G-4. Est. $3500.00-$4500.00.

Lot #331. Worth *Je Reviens* ['I Return'] smoky blue glass bottle and turquoise stopper, 3.1" [7.8 cm], the bottle entirely molded as a column with vertical ribs with steps at the top evoking a skyscraper, full and sealed, silver and blue label on front, bottom molded Lalique, in its blue box with satin lining. Utt #W-101. Est. $250.00-$350.00.

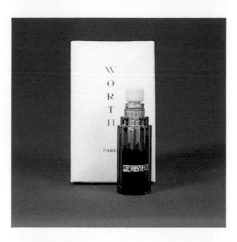

Lot #333. Worth *Requête* ['Request'] clear glass bottle and stopper, 2.9" [7.4 cm], of flat round shape with a scallop motif enameled in blue, empty, initial "W" impressed in stopper, molded Lalique. Utt #W-105 Est. $350.00-$450.00.

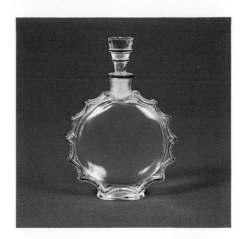

Lot #332. Worth *Projets* clear glass bottle and stopper, 2.5" [6.3 cm], the front molded with a sailboat against waves, the stopper designed as a ship's wheel, empty, with ship flag label around neck, molded signature R. Lalique. Utt #W-10. Est. $600.00-$750.00.

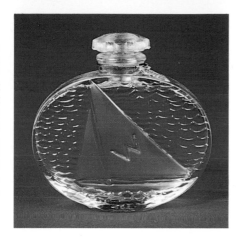

Lot #334. Maison Lalique *Baptiste* clear crystal bottle and stopper, 2.4" [6 cm], an unusual form designed with a clear perfume well and three waves of spirals above and on the stopper, bottom signed Lalique in script. Utt #CL-199. Est. $150.00-$250.00.

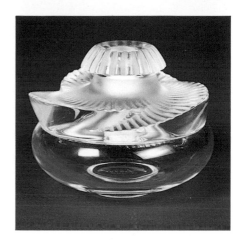

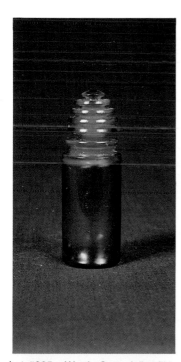

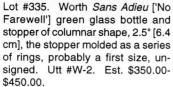

Lot #335. Worth *Sans Adieu* ['No Farewell'] green glass bottle and stopper of columnar shape, 2.5" [6.4 cm], the stopper molded as a series of rings, probably a first size, unsigned. Utt #W-2. Est. $350.00-$450.00.

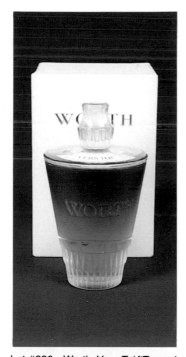

Lot #336. Worth *Vers Toi* ['Toward Thee'] clear and frosted glass bottle and stopper, 3.6" [9.1 cm], bottle of flower-pot shape embellished with rows of frosted chevrons at bottom, at the neck, and on the stopper, full and sealed, label on shoulder, molded R. Lalique on bottom, in its box; superb condition overall. Utt #W-11. Est. $600.00-$750.00.

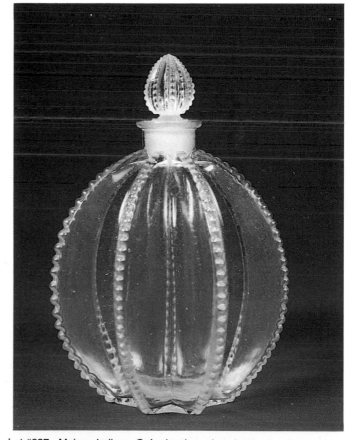

Lot #337. Maison Lalique *Grégoire* clear glass bottle and stopper, 3.9" [10 cm], with eight shell-like lobes molded with beads which beautifully combine organic and geometric motifs; bottom molded R. Lalique and also signed R. Lalique in script. Utt #ML-521. Est. $1750.00-$2250.00.

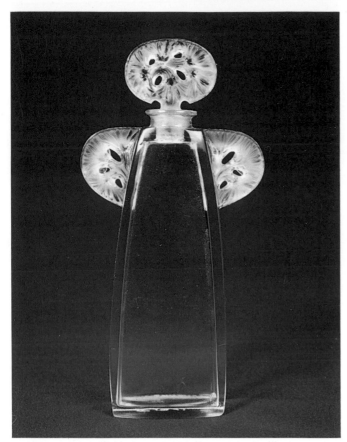

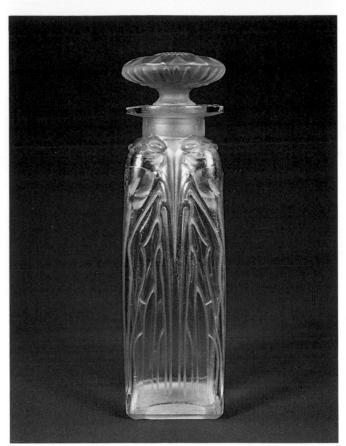

Lot #338. Maison Lalique *Anses et Bouchon Marguerite* clear and frosted glass bottle and stopper, 4.9" [12.4 cm], molded with wings of flowers with open portions, stopper similarly designed, small bruise to lip of bottle, bottom signed R. Lalique in script. Utt #ML-499. Est. $2000.00-$2500.00.

Lot #339. Maison Lalique *Les Cigales* ['The Cicadas'] clear and frosted glass bottle and stopper, 5.5" [14 cm], the bottle designed with four huge cicadas facing upward, the stopper molded as a flower, amber patina, signed R. Lalique in script on side. Utt #ML-475. Est. $3500.00-$4000.00.

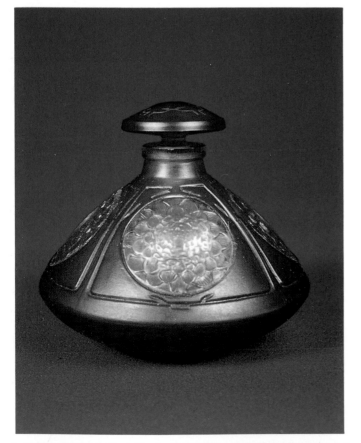

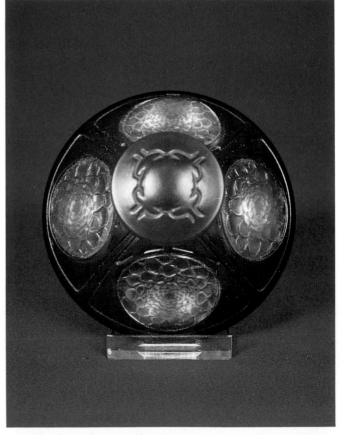

Lot #340. Maison Lalique *Quatre Soleils* ['Four Suns'] glass bottle and stopper, 2.8" [7 cm], the bottle molded on four sides with medallions which have been internally mounted with gold foil so that they appear to shine from within, covered in deep amber patina, bottom signed R. Lalique in script. This is an extremely rare and beautiful perfume bottle. Utt #ML-505. Est. $8000.00-$9500.00.

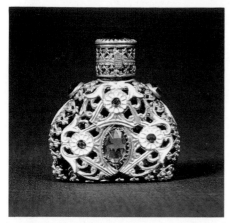

Lot #341. Clear glass bottle and cap encased in metal, 1.9" [4.8 cm], the cap mounted with a blue stone and with its dauber, bottle also mounted with blue stones and with some parts of the metal enameled white, tag on cap signed Czechoslovakia. Est. $75.00-$125.00.

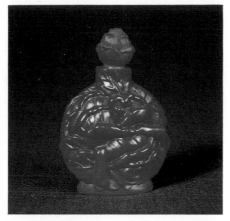

Lot #342. Miniature red opaque crystal bottle and stopper in the form of a rose in full bloom, with the stopper also in the form of a tiny rosebud, 2.4" [6 cm], with its dauber, Czech etched signature. This is a stunning miniature. Est. $250.00-$350.00.

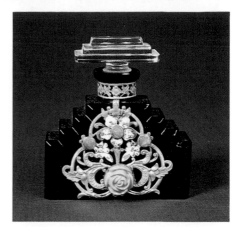

Lot #343. Black crystal bottle and clear crystal stopper, 2.8" [7.2 cm], the bottle molded with steps on each side, the stopper with a conforming design, beautiful metalwork with carved coral and green flowers, signed Czechoslovakia. Est. $300.00-$375.00.

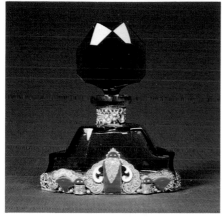

Lot #344. Smoke crystal bottle and stopper, 5" [12.5 cm], both bottle and stopper designed with large facets, the base mounted with a gold metal frame containing jewels of red opaque glass, metal collar with bow around neck, dauber lacking, signed Czechoslovakia in oval. Est. $450.00-$550.00.

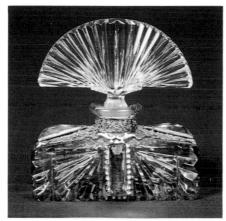

Lot #345. Peach crystal bottle and clear crystal stopper, 3.5" [8.8 cm], stopper of fan shape and cut with rays, bottle cut with facets of conforming design, metalwork with stones on shoulders of bottle and on front, dauber lacking, signed Czechoslovakia in oval [twice]. Est. $300.00-$400.00.

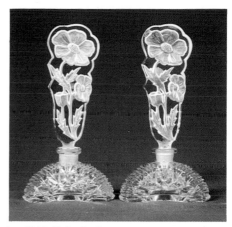

Lot #346. Pair of yellow crystal bottles and stoppers, 6.3" [16 cm], the bases highly cut on all sides, the huge stoppers intaglio cut with oriental poppies, each stopper with its dauber, Czechoslovakia in oval. Forsythe I #350. Est. $275.00-$350.00.

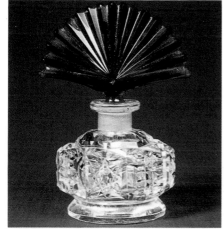

Lot #347. Clear crystal bottle and red crystal stopper, 4.9" [12.4 cm], the base cut with geometric motifs around an octagonal form, stopper designed as an opened fan, dauber lacking, signed Czechoslovakia in oval. Est. $150.00-$250.00.

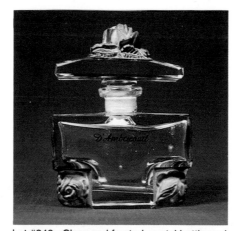

Lot #348. Clear and frosted crystal bottle and stopper, 4.9" [12.5 cm], an unusual design with roses molded on the bottom corners of the bottle and on the stopper, roses with gray and frosty white patina, the name D'Ambricourt enameled on front of the bottle, probably a commercial perfume, unsigned. Est. $350.00-$500.00.

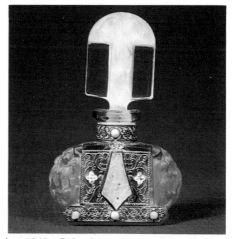

Lot #349. Pale violet crystal bottle and clear and frosted crystal stopper, 3.7" [9.5 cm], the bottle with a clear window at center and with lily of the valley on each side, conforming stopper, dauber lacking, metalwork with pearls and violet glass medallion, signed Czechoslovakia in oval. Forsythe II #943. Est. $250.00-$300.00.

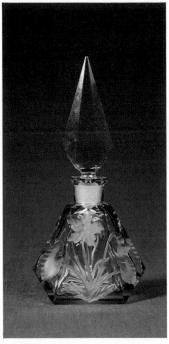

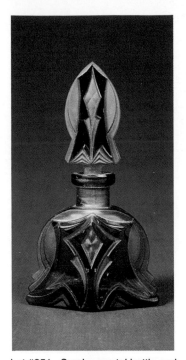

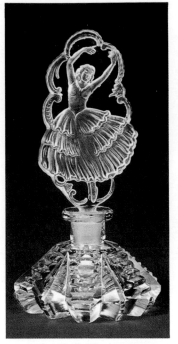

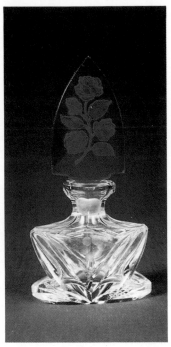

Lot #350. Violet crystal bottle and stopper, 5.5" [14 cm], the bottle intaglio cut with a design of flowers on both sides, prism stopper with its dauber, signed Czechoslovakia in oval. Est. $150.00-$225.00.

Lot #351. Smoke crystal bottle and stopper, 4.9" [12.4 cm], both bottle and stopper with identical Art Deco motifs both molded and cut, parts frosted, with its dauber, signed Czechoslovakia in oval. Est. $125.00-$200.00.

Lot #352. Clear crystal bottle and stopper, 5.7" [14.5 cm], the bottle highly cut in a star formation with step facets, the stopper intaglio cut with a dancer on point with her hands lifted gracefully over her head, [dauber lacking, thin flat chip on stopper], signed Czechoslovakia in circle. North #574. Est. $400.00-$500.00.

Lot #353. Clear crystal bottle and red crystal stopper, 5" [12.7 cm], the bottle wheel cut with a flower at center, the stopper intaglio cut with roses, with its dauber, signed Czechoslovakia in oval. Est. $150.00-$225.00.

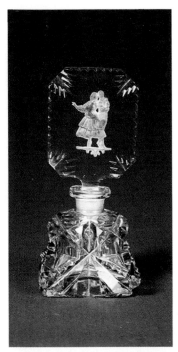

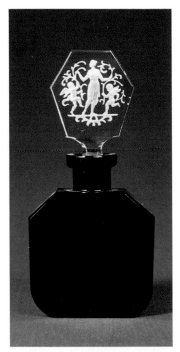

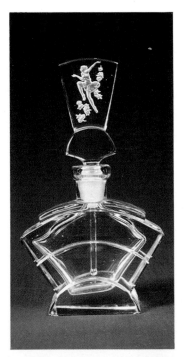

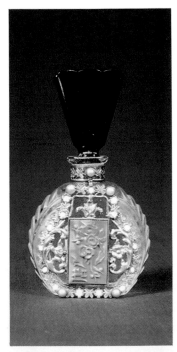

Lot #354. Lemon crystal bottle and clear crystal stopper, 5.4" [13.7 cm], the base highly cut and intricately faceted, the stopper intaglio cut with a pair of Spanish dancers, with its dauber, signed Czechoslovakia in oval. Est. $250.00-$350.00.

Lot #355. Black crystal bottle and clear crystal stopper, 5.7" [14.5 cm], the bottle basically rectangular but with faceted shoulders, the stopper intaglio cut with a Grecian goddess and two winged cupids surrounded by branches, with its dauber, undoubtedly a Hoffman design, unsigned. Est. $400.00-$500.00.

Lot #356. Yellow crystal bottle and stopper, 5.4" [13.7 cm], bottle molded with curved steps, stopper mirrors the bottle design and is intaglio cut with a leaping dancer and flowers, with its dauber, signed Czechoslovakia in circle. Est. $300.00-$400.00.

Lot #357. Clear and frosted crystal bottle and black glass stopper, 4.2" [10.7 cm], the front of the bottle covered with metalwork having pearls and a large jade glass medallion with Chinese symbols, black glass stopper in a fan shape and with dauber, signed Czechoslovakia in oval. North #54. Est. $300.00-$400.00.

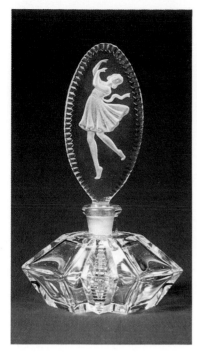

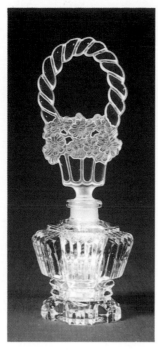

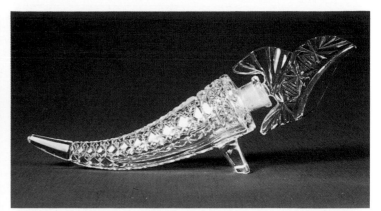

Lot #360. Clear crystal bottle and stopper in the shape of a scimitar, 9.5" [24.1 cm], base highly cut in a star pattern, conforming stopper of semi-tiara shape, with dauber, signed Czechoslovakia in oval and in circle. Est. $300.00-$450.00.

Lot #358. Clear crystal bottle and stopper, 5.9" [15 cm], the base with multiple facets, the stopper intaglio cut with a ballerina, scalloped edges to stopper and on front of bottle, with its dauber, signed Czechoslovakia in oval. North #220 [stopper]. Est. $400.00-$500.00.

Lot #359. Clear crystal bottle and stopper, 7.6" [19.3 cm], the bottom pressed rather than cut into a six-sided urn, the stopper molded as a basket with tall handle overflowing with flowers, with its dauber, the base molded Czechoslovakia. Est. $150.00-$200.00.

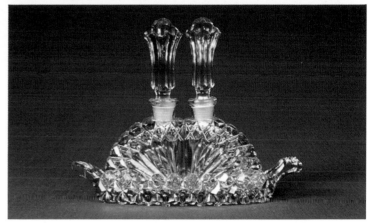

Lot #361. Pair of unusual peach crystal bottles and stoppers [daubers lacking], each 4.6" [11.7 cm], in their highly cut and faceted boat-shaped carrier, each bottle signed Czechoslovakia. Three-piece set. Est. $200.00-$250.00.

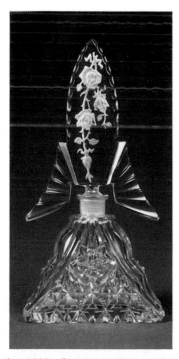

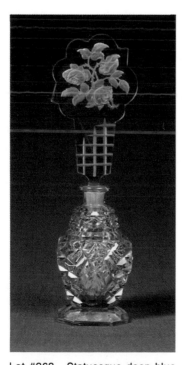

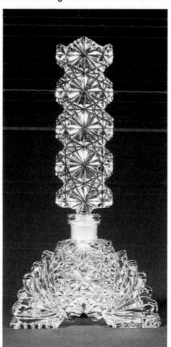

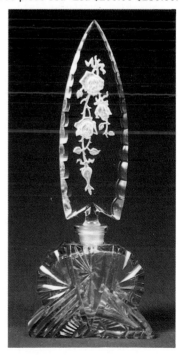

Lot #362. Statuesque blue crystal bottle and stopper, 9" [22.9 cm], the bottle of triangular form with many facets, the stopper a beautiful tiara intaglio cut with roses and scalloped on edges, with its dauber, signed Czechoslovakia in line. Est. $500.00-$650.00.

Lot #363. Statuesque deep blue crystal bottle and stopper, 9.1" [23 cm], the bottle highly faceted on four sides, the stopper intaglio cut with roses, dauber lacking, signed Czechoslovakia in oval [twice]; this color could be called "Ingrid Blue" as it is much deeper than normal. Est. $500.00-$650.00.

Lot #364. Statuesque clear crystal bottle and stopper, 9.2" [23.4 cm], the bottle resting on two feet and cut with rays and stars, stopper wholly cut with stars, with its dauber but with bruise on inner tongue of stopper, signed Czechoslovakia in circle and with silver label. Est. $375.00-$475.00.

Lot #365. Statuesque blue crystal bottle and clear crystal stopper, 9.5" [24.1 cm], the base cut asymmetrically with pleats and rays, the stopper shaped as an arrow and intaglio cut with roses, with its dauber, signed Czechoslovakia in oval. Est. $450.00-$550.00.

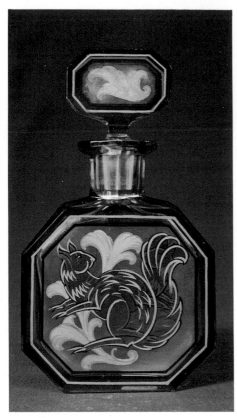

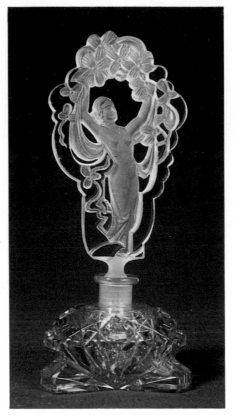

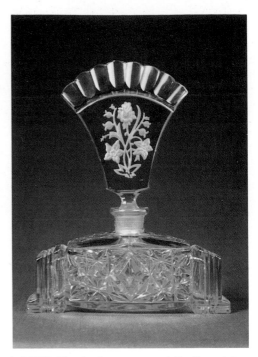

Lot #366. Unusual amber crystal cologne bottle and stopper, 7.3" [18.5 cm], both of octagonal form, a squirrel and stylized leaves enameled in green, black, and orange on both sides of bottle and on stopper, unsigned; no similar example in published sources. Est. $400.00-$500.00.

Lot #367. Blue crystal bottle and stopper, 8.2" [20.8 cm], the base highly cut, stopper molded with a lady holding a garland of flowers aloft, intricate cut-outs on stopper [dauber lacking], signed Czechoslovakia and with silver label. North #307 [stopper]. Est. $600.00-$750.00.

Lot #368. Massive lime green crystal bottle and stopper, 7.5" [19 cm], the base of oblong shape resting on two feet, the stopper of fan shape intaglio cut with flowers, with its dauber, signed Czechoslovakia in circle. Est. $350.00-$450.00.

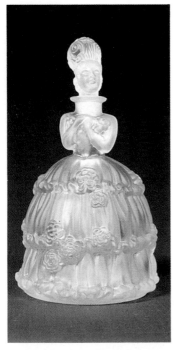

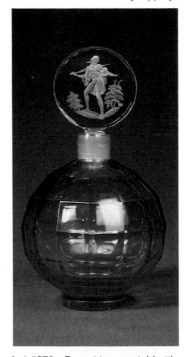

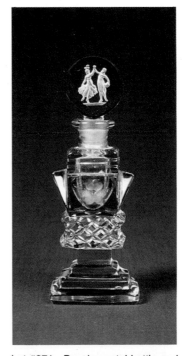

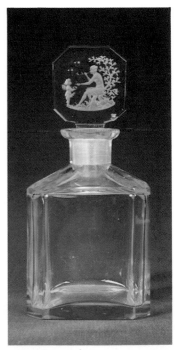

Lot #369. Frosted crystal bottle and stopper, 6" [15.2 cm], molded entirely as an 18th century lady with tall wig and flowered dress, amber patina, unsigned. North #367. Est. $200.00-$300.00.

Lot #370. Deep blue crystal bottle and stopper, 6.2" [15.8 cm], in the shape of a globe with pedestal base, the surface of the globe covered with geometric facets, stopper intaglio cut with a man playing the violin against a background of trees, by Hoffman, signed with the Ingrid butterfly. Est. $400.00-$500.00.

Lot #371. Peach crystal bottle and stopper, 5" [12.7 cm], the bottle on a pedestal cut with many motifs and having a small interior well for the perfume, stopper intaglio cut with a pair of dancers, dauber lacking, signed Czechoslovakia in oval. Forsythe II, #881. Est. $150.00-$200.00.

Lot #372. Aqua crystal bottle and stopper, 6.9" [17.5 cm], the bottle of square decanter form, the stopper beautifully cut with Cupid holding a bowl from which his mother, Venus, blows bubbles of love, signed with the Hoffman butterfly on the stopper, bottom also acid signed and with rare Hoffman paper label. Est. $450.00-$600.00.

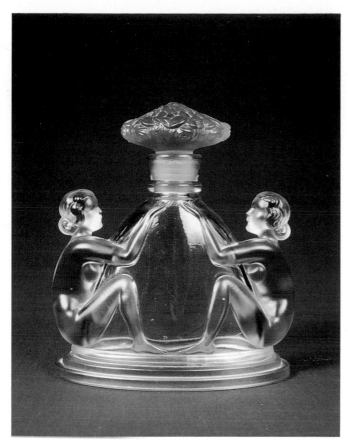

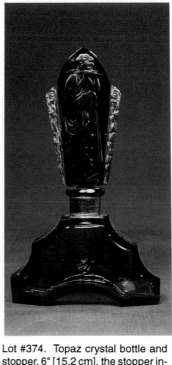

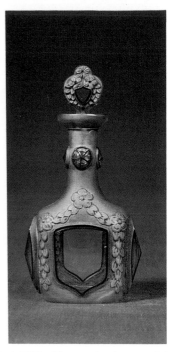

Lot #373. Rare amber crystal bottle and stopper, 5.2" [13.2 cm], designed as two nudes encircling an urn, stopper molded as a bouquet of flowers, stopper without dauber, unsigned. North #590; Forsythe II #727. Est. $800.00-$1000.00.

Lot #374. Topaz crystal bottle and stopper, 6" [15.2 cm], the stopper intaglio cut with a dancing nude playing the flute, base with broad facets on two feet, with its dauber, bottom signed Czechoslovakia and Ingrid. North #406. Est. $600.00-$750.00.

Lot #375. Very early clear crystal bottle and stopper, 5.2" [13.2 cm], the bottle with a shield-form window front and back surmounted by garlands of flowers, oval faceted windows on the sides of the bottle and on four sides around neck, stopper also with clear window and flowers, brown patina and black enamel detail, prob. for commercial use, signed Czechoslovakia in line. Est. $400.00-$500.00.

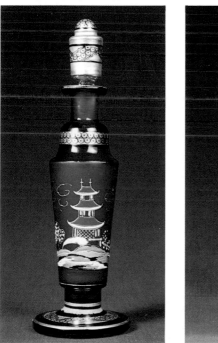

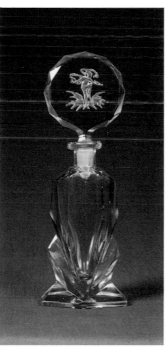

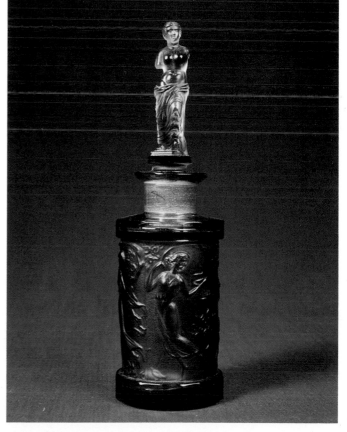

Lot #376. Cobalt blue glass cologne bottle and clear glass stopper, 8.3" [21 cm], decorated with an oriental scene and Pagoda enameled in multicolor, gold and black enamel decoration on pedestal base and on stopper; country of origin undetermined, but probably Czechoslovakia. Est. $150.00-$200.00.

Lot #377. Tall and elegant blue crystal bottle and stopper, 7.8" [19.8 cm], the bottle cut with large angular facets, the stopper intaglio cut with a scarf dancer and with a faceted border, with its very long dauber, unsigned. Est. $350.00-$450.00.

Lot #378. Violet crystal bottle and stopper, 6.3" [16 cm], the bottle with a frieze of classical dancers, the top molded as the *Venus de Milo*, with its violet dauber, unsigned, designed by Hoffman. Forsythe II #928. Est. $600.00-$700.00.

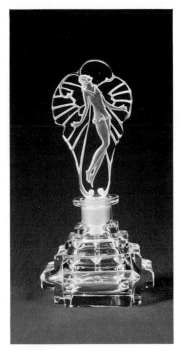

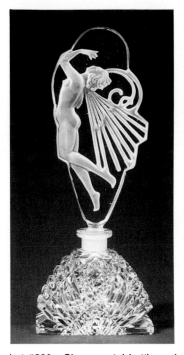

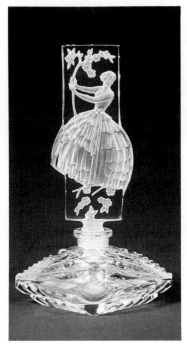

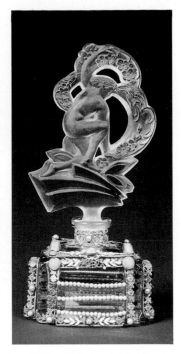

Lot #379. Clear crystal bottle and stopper, 5.7" [14.5 cm], the bottle shaped as a four-sided pyramid with steps, the stopper intaglio cut with an Art Deco lady with butterfly wings, with its dauber. North #575. Est. $400.00-$500.00.

Lot #380. Clear crystal bottle and stopper, 8.8" [22.4 cm], the base highly cut with pleats and rays, the huge stopper intaglio cut with a nude butterfly-woman, dauber lacking, signed Czechoslovakia in line. North #365. Est. $700.00-$850.00.

Lot #381. Clear crystal bottle and stopper, 6.2" [15.7 cm], the base highly cut and of an irregular hexagonal form, the stopper intaglio cut with a lady in a full gown apparently swinging from a branch, dauber lacking, signed Czechoslovakia in oval. North #390. Est. $500.00-$600.00.

Lot #382. Pink crystal bottle and frosted glass stopper, 6.9" [17.5 cm], the bottle with rectangular step motifs and covered with metalwork mounted with pearls and carved pink stones, stopper molded as a nude holding garlands of flowers, dauber lacking, signed Czechoslovakia in oval [twice]; this stopper is rare. Est. $600.00-$750.00.

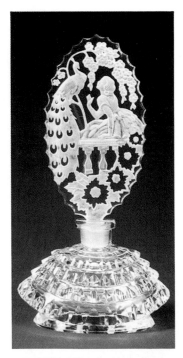

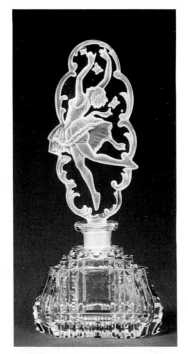

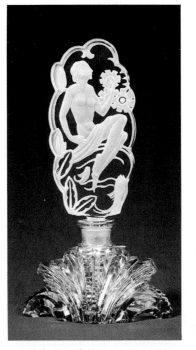

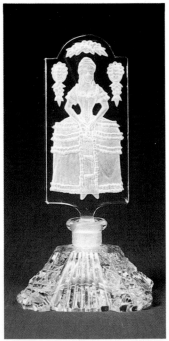

Lot #383. Clear crystal bottle and light blue stopper, 6.9" [17.5 cm], the base having a skirt-like appearance made by rows of scalloped facets, the stopper with scalloped edges and intaglio cut with a lady and a peacock in a bower of flowers, dauber lacking, signed Czechoslovakia in circle and with Morlee label. North #369. Est. $400.00-$550.00.

Lot #384. Yellow crystal bottle and clear crystal stopper, 7" [17.8 cm], the base highly cut with a central window and framed by rows of lines, the stopper intaglio cut with a ballerina and molded with scallops, dauber lacking, signed Czechoslovakia in oval. North #164 (stopper). Est. $500.00-$600.00.

Lot #385. Large lemon crystal bottle and stopper, 6.8" [17.2 cm], the base highly cut with lines and facets, the stopper intaglio cut with a nude supported as if on waves and with fish near the bottom, leaves and flowers in the Art Deco style, [dauber lacking], signed Czechoslovakia in circle. Forsythe II #732. Est. $550.00-$650.00.

Lot #386. Clear crystal bottle and crystal stopper, 6.6" [16.8 cm], the bottle with four sides and highly cut on each, the stopper intaglio cut with an 18th century lady in formal gown having a wide bustle on both sides, with dauber, base signed Czechoslovakia in circle. North #229 (stopper). Est. $500.00-$600.00.

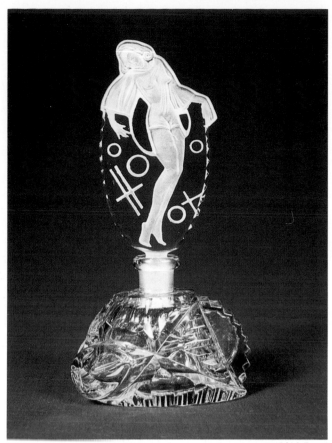

Lot #387. Yellow crystal bottle and clear crystal stopper, 6.5" [16.5 cm], the bottle molded in an angular, asymmetrical form, the stopper molded and intaglio cut in the shape of a dancer in a short, transparent garment, dauber lacking, signed Czechoslovakia in oval. Est. $500.00-$650.00.

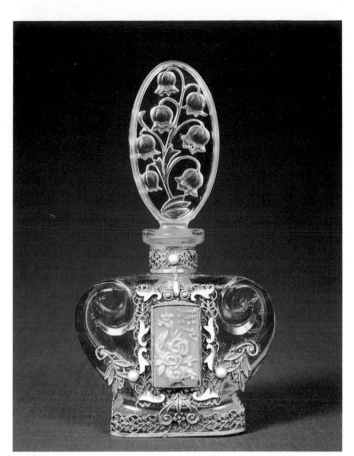

Lot #388. Green crystal bottle and stopper, 5.7" [14.5 cm], the stopper with lily of the valley intaglio cut, the bottle of heart shape with metalwork and a green glass medallion molded with flowers and Chinese characters, with its dauber, signed Czechoslovakia in oval. Est. $400.00-$500.00.

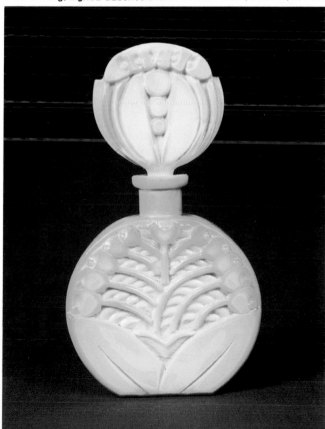

Lot #389. Aqua opaque crystal bottle and stopper, 5.2" [13.2 cm], both sides of the bottle molded with flowers highly stylized in the Art Deco manner, stopper with a similar molded design on one side, dauber lacking, unsigned; this is a rare design and color. Est. $700.00-$850.00.

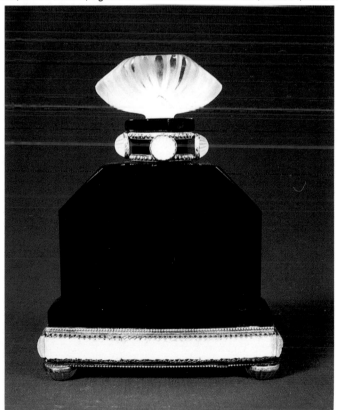

Lot #390. Black crystal bottle and clear and frosted stopper, 5.5" [14 cm], the stopper with a dauber as a nude with upward flowing hair, the neck and the base with metalwork embellished with ribbed cabochons and frosted glass panels of flowers [three panels with apparent fractures in the identical place], metal signed Austria. This rare and elegant bottle is one of the finest designed by Hoffman. Est. $3000.00-$3500.00.

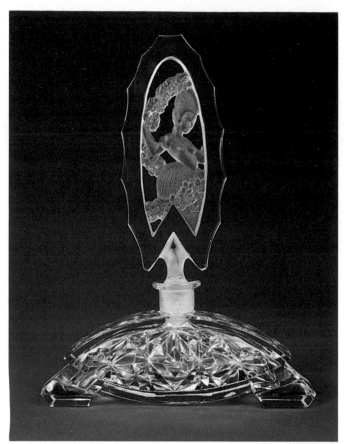

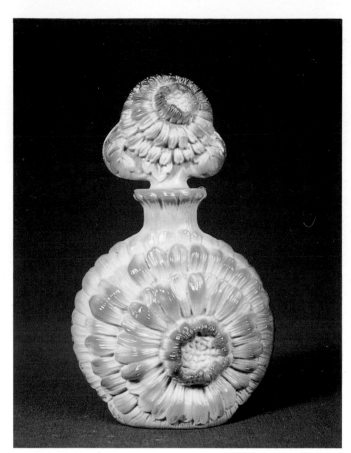

Lot #391. Fine large clear crystal bottle and stopper, 8.5" [21.6 cm], the highly faceted base resting on bilateral feet, stopper with scalloped edges and molded with an elegant lady in a transparent dress amid flower garlands, with dauber, signed Czechoslovakia. Est. $500.00-$600.00.

Lot #392. Malachite glass bottle and stopper, 5.7" [14.4 cm], the bottle molded on both sides as a single open chrysanthemum, the stopper with the same design on a smaller scale, dauber lacking, unsigned. North #814. Est. $500.00-$650.00.

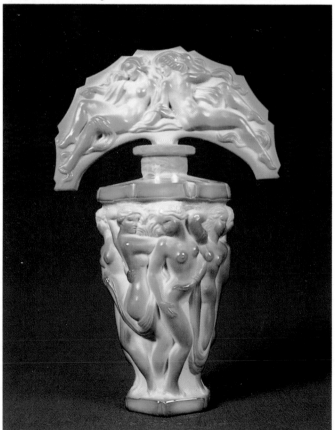

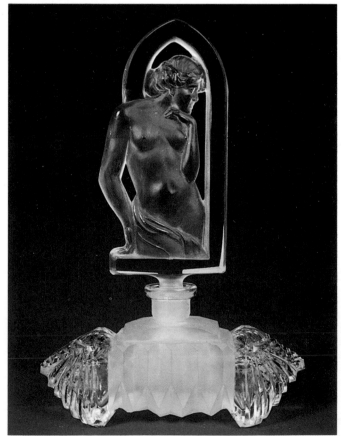

Lot #393. Malachite glass perfume bottle and stopper, 7" [17.8 cm], the bottle molded with intertwined nudes, tiara stopper with two nudes, dauber lacking, signed Czechoslovakia in circle; this bottle has very beautiful mold and color variation. North back cover #A. Est. $1000.00-$1250.00.

Lot #394. Rare clear and frosted crystal bottle and stopper, 7.2" [18.3 cm], the elongated base highly faceted, the stopper beautifully molded with a nude woman framed by a window [dauber lacking], unsigned. North #364. Est. $1000.00-$1200.00.

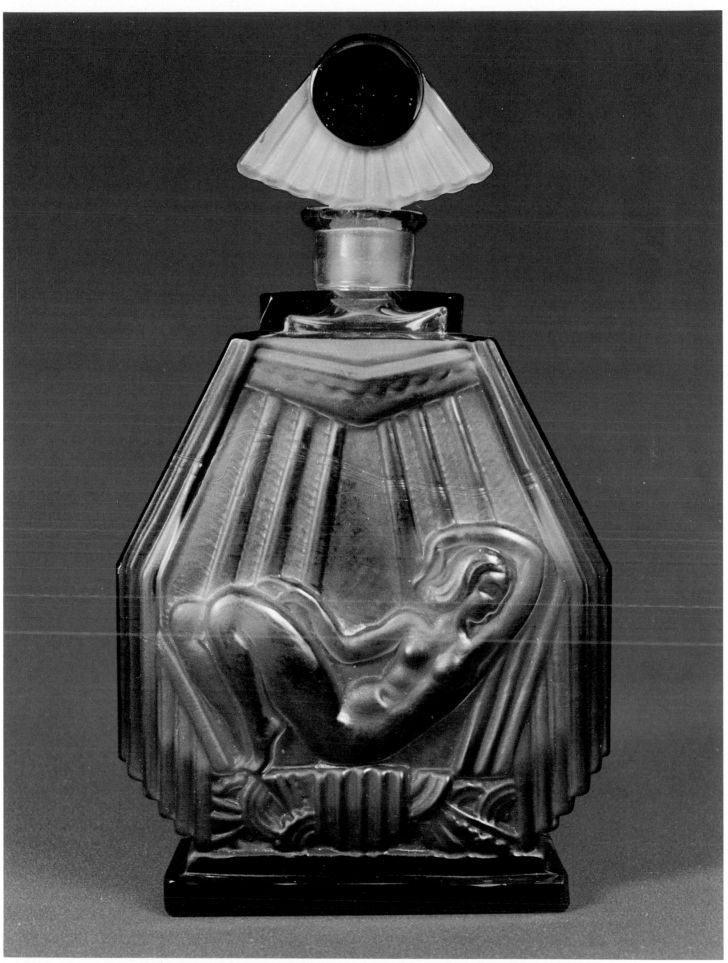

Lot #395. Fine quality amber crystal bottle and stopper, 8" [20.3 cm], the bottle designed by Hoffman in the 1920's Art Deco style with a nude across the bottle surrounded by drapery, the stopper with an Egyptian sunray motif, unsigned. Est. $1750.00-$2000.00.

The Crowned-Heads of Perfume

Les Têtes Couronnées du Parfum

Rodney L. Baer

This article is dedicated to Pauline de Morcia,
who has always shared her love of crown-tops and of collecting.

Cet article est dédié à Pauline de Morcia qui a toujours partagé
son amour de la collection et des flacons à bouchon en couronne

The use of figural porcelain containers for perfume has a long history. Marvelous early examples were made by the Meissen factories in Germany in the late 18th century and throughout the next hundred years. These miniature sculpture-like flacons often held a surprise element of humor. An excellent example is a very old Meissen bottle shaped like a monk carrying a sheaf of wheat [cf. Martin 1982, p. 13]. Upon removing the monk's head stopper, it is revealed that a girl has been hidden within the sheaf of wheat. Building upon this long tradition of humorous porcelain figural bottles are the crown-top perfume bottles. From the late 1800's through the 1930's, crown-top figural perfume bottles were made by many German factories. The hundreds, maybe even thousands, of different shapes make collecting crown-tops an exciting challenge for the perfume bottle fancier.

Most of the crown-top bottles were sold empty and ready to hold the buyer's favorite scent, but occasionally, examples are found with labels and packaging indicating that crown-tops were used by commercial perfume companies to enhance the marketing of their product. The "cute" factor leads one to think that the target consumer of these bottles might have been young women and girls. The typical stopper, which gives these bottle their name, is shaped like a crown. The stopper, with a cork fitting, is of two-piece construction that allows the bottle to be opened and closed by turning the crown a half twist. This shaker style is the most common type of stopper, but other types are also found. Solid crowns and solid flower shaped stoppers with cork fittings are also seen. In some cases, the entire crown screws off leaving a tiny spout in the cork fitting. The band above the cork fitting often is marked Germany or has a decorative pattern. Occasionally, a company name will be molded on the band.

The vast majority of crown-top perfumes were made in Germany and Bavaria. Other examples can be found from France, Holland, Austria, England, and Japan. The German

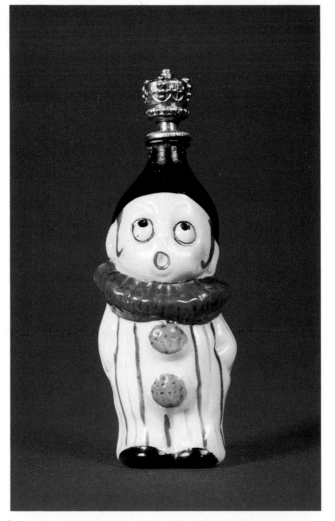

Figure 1. A baby Pierrot is singing. All of the perfume bottles photographed for this article are from the Collection of Rodney L. Baer and Randall B. Monsen.

L'utilisation de figurines de porcelaine pour contenir du parfum a une bien longue histoire. Parmi les plus vieilles sont des exemples faits à Meissen en Allemagne à la fin du XVIIème et le siècle suivant. Ces flacons que l'on croirait sculptés recellaient souvent un élément d'humour. Un exemple excellent est un vieux flacon de Meissen d'un moine portant une gerbe de blé [voir Martin 1982, p.13]. En enlevant le bouchon (la tête du moine) l'on découvre qu'il y a une jeune femme cachée dans la gerbe de blé. Les bouchons de parfum en forme de couronne continuent cette longue tradition de flacons figuratifs en porcelaine. De la fin du XIXème jusqu'aux années 30, des usines allemandes fabriquaient des flacons de parfum figuratifs en porcelaine avec des bouchons en couronne. Les centaines, voir les milliers, de formes différentes rendent la collection de bouchons en couronne un défi pour le collectionneur de flacons de parfum.

La plupart des flacons avec des bouchons en couronne étaient vendus vides prêts à recevoir le parfum préféré de l'acheteur; mais parfois on trouve des exemples avec des étiquettes et un emballage démontrant que les bouchons en couronne étaient utilisés par les fabricants de parfums pour améliorer les ventes de leur produit. Le bouchon typique, dont est dérivé le nom, ressemble à une couronne. Le bouchon avec une pièce en liège, est une construction en deux pièces qui permet d'ouvrir et de fermer le flacon en donnant un demi tour au bouchon. Ce style shaker est le type de bouchon le plus répandu, mais il en existe d'autres. Des bouchons massifs en forme de couronne ou de fleurs avec des pièces en liège existent aussi. Dans certains cas, la couronne entière se dévisse laissant un petit versoir dans la pièce de liège. L'anneau au-dessus de la pièce de liège porte souvent la marque "Germany" ou un motif décoratif. Parfois l'anneau portera le nom de la société.

La vaste majorité des flacons à bouchon en

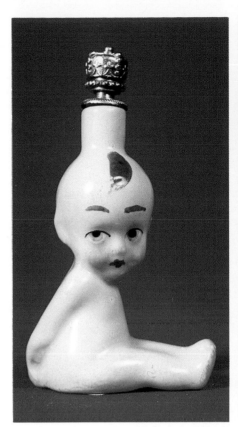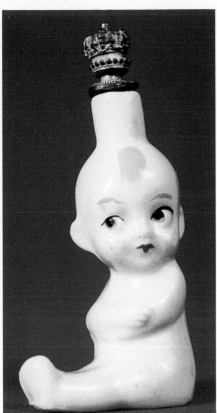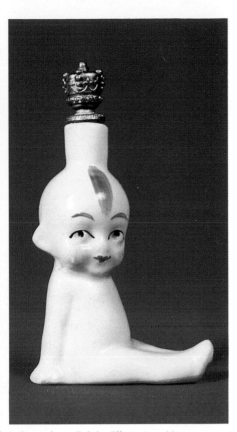

Figures 2, 3, 4. The Baby Kewpies. In each of the five known examples, the arms and hands are in a slightly different position.

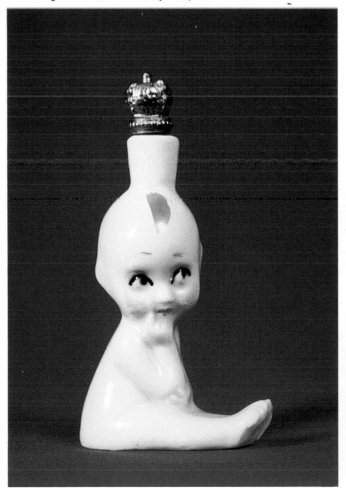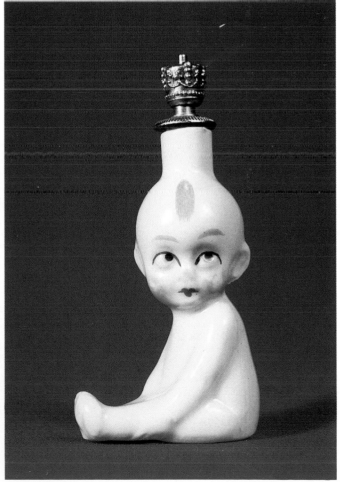

Figures 5, 6. Baby Kewpies.

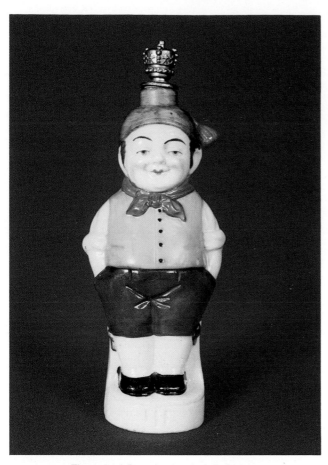

Figure 7. A Bavarian boy in lederhosen.

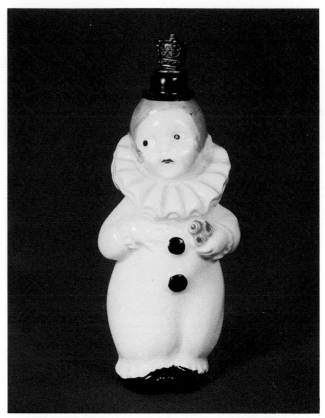

Figure 8. A baby clown holding roses, marked Bavaria.

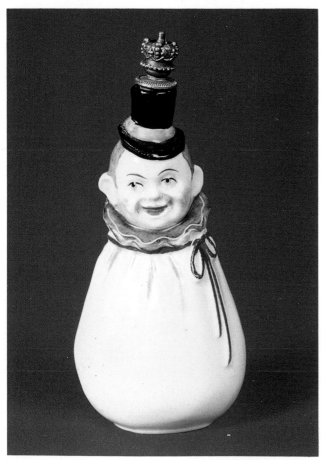

Figure 9. A boy in a bag, marked Germany.

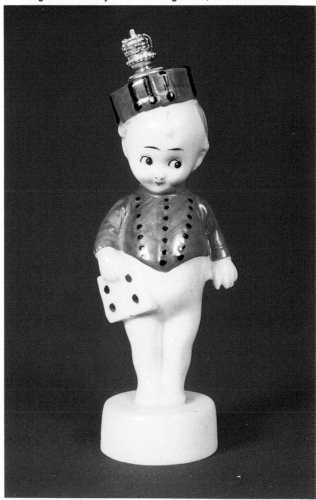

Figure 10. A Bellhop with loveletter; this model is by Goebel.

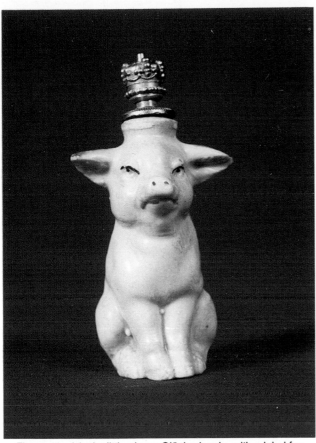

Figure 11. A lucky little pig, or Glückschwein, with a label for commercial perfume underneath.

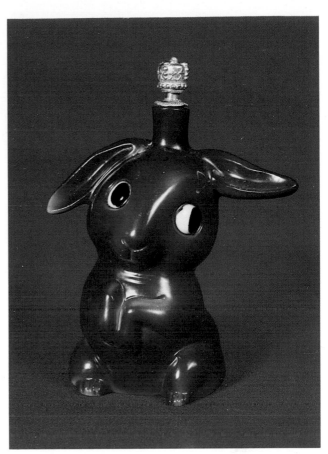

Figure 12. A Rabbit, in brilliant cobalt blue, by Goebel.

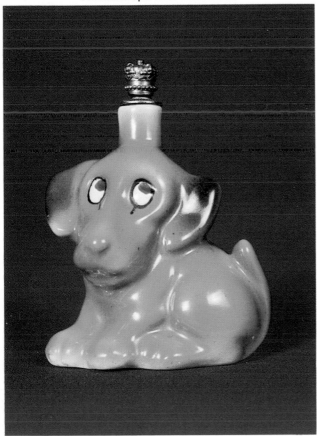

Figure 13. A Dachshund, in green, by Goebel.

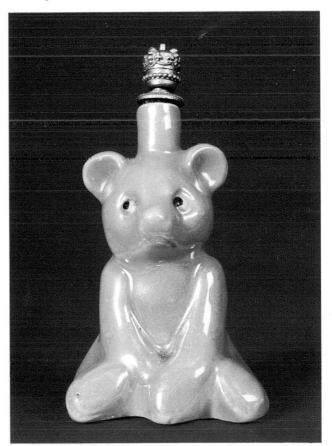

Figure 14. A Teddy Bear, looking very pensive.

examples are marked in a variety of ways. Many can be found with inked bottom stamps that say Germany, Bavaria, Made in Germany, or sometimes even the company that imported or distributed the bottle. These inked marks were not always indelible, so sometimes they are very faint or completely erased. Impressed marks were also used. Germany is often found impressed on the back or side of the bottle and is sometimes accompanied by impressed numbers. These impressed numbers appear to have been mold numbers and may sometimes be the only identifying mark found on the bottle. Beautiful

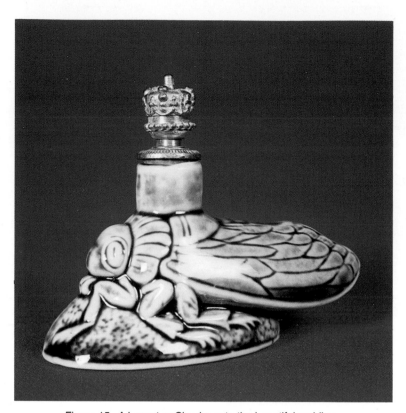

Figure 15. A Locust or Cicada; note the beautiful molding.

examples also exist with absolutely no identifying marks, adding to the mystery of collecting.

Several major porcelain factories made crown-top bottles and used their company mark to identify them. The Sitzendorf, Schneider, Schafer & Vater, and Goebel porcelain companies all manufactured crown-top bottles. The crown-tops of the Goebel Company are particularly popular

couronne viennent d'Allemagne et de la Bavière, mais il y en a de France, des Pays-Bas, de l'Autriche, du Royaume-Uni et du Japon. Les exemples allemands portent différentes marques. Beaucoup ont des marques en encre sur leur base avec "Germany" "Bavaria" "Made in Germany" ou parfois le nom de la société qui importait ou diffusait les flacons. Ces marques n'étaient pas toujours indélébiles, ce qui explique qu'elles sont parfois difficiles à lire ou absentes. Il y a aussi des marques en relief. "Germany" est souvent en relief sur le dos ou sur le côté du flacon, parfois accompagné de chiffres. Ces chiffres en relief semblent avoir été des numéros de moules et sont parfois les seules indications d'origine sur le flacon. De très beaux exemples existent qui ne portent aucune marque, ce qui ne fait qu'accentuer le mystère qui accompagne l'art du collectionneur.

Plusieurs maisons de porcelaine importantes faisaient des flacons à bouchon en couronne et utilisaient

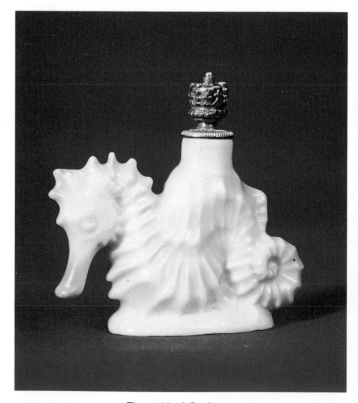

Figure 16. A Seahorse.

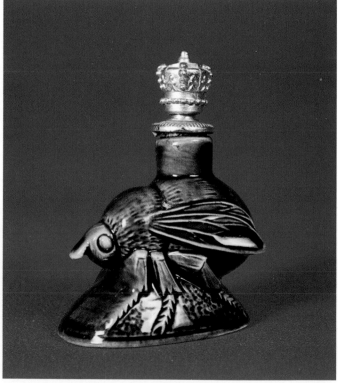

Figure 17. A Housefly, very fat it seems.

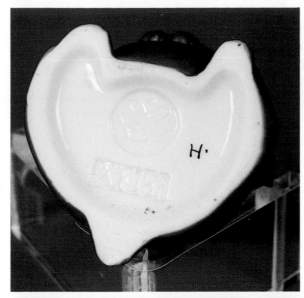

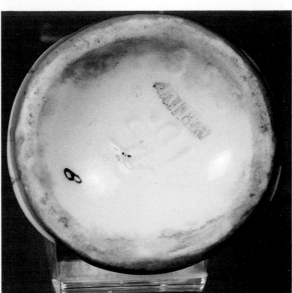

Figure 18 [Left]. Goebel molded mark of a crown over WG, with mold numbers and artist's initial; bottle is from Fig. 12.

Figure 19 [Right]. Different Goebel marking, bottle in Fig. 33, also marked Germany in black ink and with artist's initial.

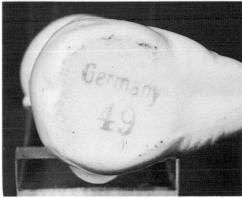

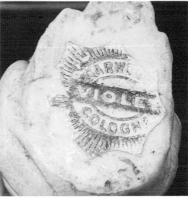

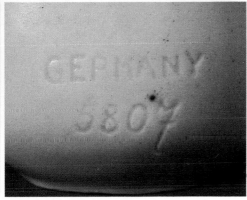

Figure 20. 'Germany 49' stamped in red ink on the bottom of a Kewpie, from Fig. 2.

Figure 21. The pig in Fig. 11 with paper label for Violet cologne.

Figure 22. The back side of the bottle in Fig. 9; the numbers identify this particular model.

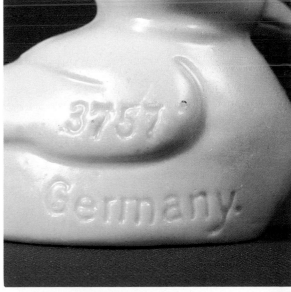

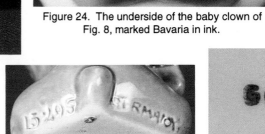

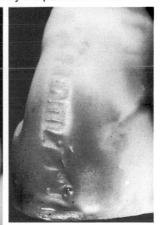

Figure 24. The underside of the baby clown of Fig. 8, marked Bavaria in ink.

Figure 25. The back of a small dog; 'Germany' carved into the mold straight up the dog's back.

Figure 23. The Canary, Fig. 40, model #'s molded.

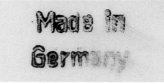

Figure 26. One type of common inkstamp.

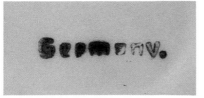

Figure 27. Molded inscriptions on the back of the dog, Fig. 41.

Figure 28. Germany stamped in red ink, easily washed off.

among collectors. They are especially well-marked, including extensive mold numbers and the crown mark that was used between 1935 and 1942. The quality of the Goebel bottles is usually exceptional with wonderful humor and great detail.

A collector of crown-tops might be a generalist, collecting the wide variety of shapes available, or a specialist, specializing in a specific category. Clowns and Pierrots, Oriental, Egyptian, and other ethnic figures, children, and historical ladies are some of the categories that might interest the collector of human figurals. For the animal fancier, crown-tops represent a veritable zoo of possibilities including dogs, cats, birds, insects, elephants, camels, bears, and lions. Crown-tops in the shape of flower baskets and vases of flowers are another possibility. Art Deco enthusiasts will find many ex-

leur marque afin de les identifier. Les maisons Sitzendorf, Schneider, Schafer & Vater, et Goebel fabriquaient toutes des flacons à bouchon en couronne. Les flacons à bouchon en couronne de la société Goebel sont particulièrement populaires auprès des collectionneurs. Ils sont bien marqués, comprenant des numéros de moule détaillés et la marque en couronne utilisée de 1935 à 1942. La qualité des flacons Goebel est exceptionnelle pour son humour et ses nombreux détails.

Un collectionneur de flacons à bouchon en couronne peut décider d'être éclectique, recherchant toutes les formes disponibles ou d'être spécialiste choisissant une catégorie particulière. Clowns et Pierrots, figures orientales, égyptiennes et d'autres figures ethniques, figures féminines et enfantines empruntées à l'histoire sont quelques-unes des catégories

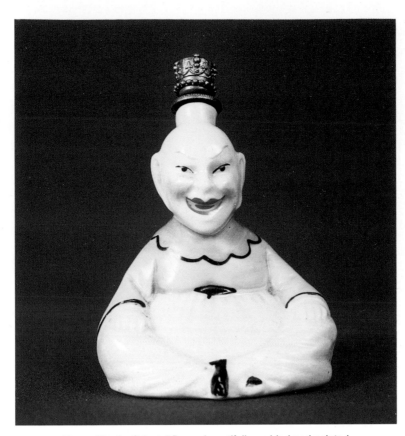

Figure 29. An Oriental figure, beautifully molded and painted.

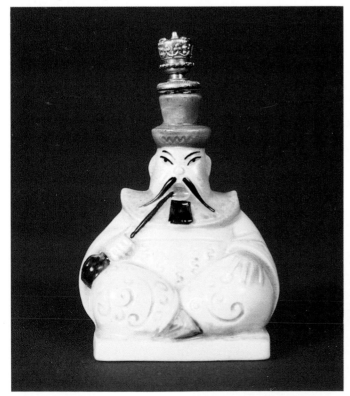

Figure 30. A Turkish potentate with a long pipe.

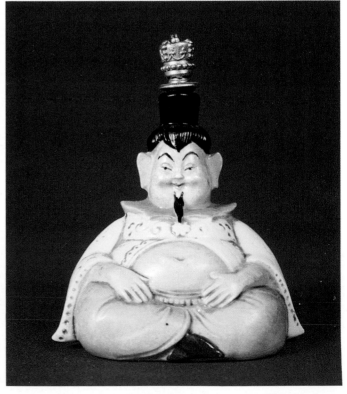

Figure 31. An Oriental figure of impressive girth.

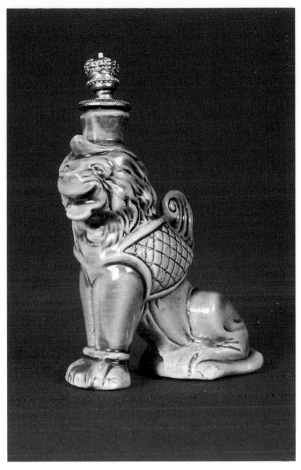

Figure 32. A laughing Lion.

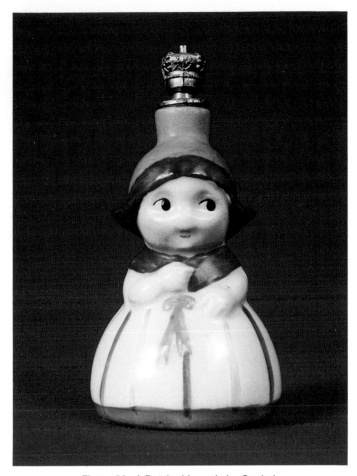

Figure 33. A Dutch girl, made by Goebel.

amples with wonderful deco style [Monsen and Baer 1995 - Lot #113]. One small group of crown-tops are shaped like Kewpie babies. Similar to the Kewpie doll designed and patontod in 1913 by Rose O'Neill, but without the blue wings, these little bottles are favorites among collectors. There are known to be five different poses for this Kewpie bottle - hands by the legs, arms crossed behind the back, hand under the chin, arms crossed on chest, and arms down by the sides. The subtle differences of these poses make this a difficult set to put together and the possibility of finding yet another pose enlivens the adventure of collecting.

Originally sold

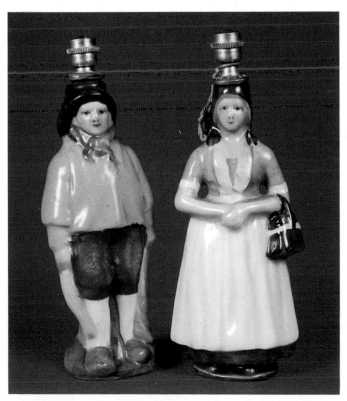

Figure 34. A Dutch fisherman and his wife, made in Holland.

qui peuvent intéresser un collectionneur de figurines à formes humaines. Pour ceux qui aiment les animaux, les flacons à bouchon en couronne constituent un peuple animal complet comprenant des chiens, des chats, des oiseaux, des insectes, des éléphants, des chameaux, des ours et des lions. On trouve aussi des paniers et des vases de fleurs. Les amateurs d'Art Déco trouveront de nombreuses pièces très belles [Monsen and Baer 1995 - lot 113]. Une petite catégorie de flacons à bouchon en couronne est celle des poupées Kewpie. Bien aimées par les collectionneurs, elles ressemblent à la poupée Kewpie conçue et brevetée par Rose O'Neill, mais elles n'en ont pas les ailes bleues. Cinq poses différentes sont connues pour ce flacon Kewpie - mains à côté des jambes, bras croisés derrière le dos, main sous le menton, bras croisés devant et les bras le long du

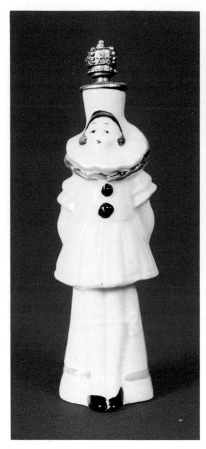

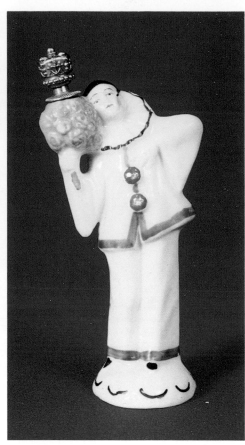

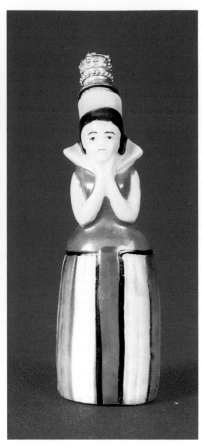

Figure 35. Pierrette beautifully molded and with large ruffle.

Figure 36. A beautifully molded Pierrot, with a bouquet of flowers.

Figure 37. A slender lady in bright Art Deco costume.

as novelties, crown-top perfume bottles probably sold for a few pennies. The throw-away nature of these bottles has added to their present rarity. The collector today can expect to pay from slightly under one hundred dollars for more common examples to several hundred dollars for very fine examples. As with all perfume bottles, condition is very important. Collectors look for examples with good mold, nicely detailed painting, no damage, and the crown. While the crown-top stopper is an essential part, one should never turn down an interesting bottle merely for the lack of it.

Like all areas of perfume bottle collecting, one category leads to another. The collector of crown-top porcelain bottles might soon also acquire a few of the German glass bottles, made of mercury glass or of milk-white glass or of clear glass with swirls of color. These are usually found with a mercury glass stopper shaped as a glass ball with dauber, but occasionally they have the typical metal crown-top stopper. Another type of glass bottle with a crown top is the googlie-eyed face made of thin milk glass [Monsen and Baer 1992 - Lot #87]. Figural bottles that incorporate the stopper in the design [Monsen and Baer 1992 - Lots # 89 - #93] are also natural "case mates" with crown-tops. There are few people who can look upon a grouping of crown-top perfumes without smiling at these "scents of humor".

References:
Martin, Hazel. *Figural Perfume and Scent Bottles.* Lancaster, CA: Hazel Martin, 1982.
Farnsworth, Craig & Helen. Crown Tops. *Perfume and Scent Bottle News*, Vol 4, #3, April, 1992.

corps. Les différences subtiles de ces poses rendent difficile la constitution d'un groupe et la possibilité de trouver encore une autre pose donne du piment à l'aventure de la collection.

Vendus à l'origine comme des bibelots, les flacons à bouchon en couronne étaient probablement vendus pour quelques centimes. La nature éphémère des ces flacons a contribué à leur rareté actuelle. Le collectionneur peut s'attendre à devoir payer les exemples courants un peu moins de 100 dollars et plusieurs centaines pour de beaux exemples. Avec tous les flacons de parfum, l'état est très important. Les collectionneurs cherchent des exemples bien moulés, avec de bons détails dans la peinture, pas de dégâts et la couronne. Quoique le bouchon soit une pièce essentielle, on ne devrait jamais refuser un flacon intéressant simplement parce que le bouchon manque.

Ici, comme dans d'autres domaines de la collection de flacons de parfum, une catégorie en appelle souvent une autre. Le collectionneur de flacons à bouchon en couronne achetera un jour quelques flacons en verre allemands, faits de verre mercure et de verre transparent avec des spirales en couleur. Ceux-ci sont souvent assortis d'un bouchon en verre mercure en forme d'une boule de verre avec un applicateur, mais parfois ils ont un bouchon classique en couronne en métal. Un autre type de flacon à bouchon en couronne est le visage aux yeux ébahis fait en opaline fine [Monsen and Baer 1992 - lot 87]. Des flacons à figurine dont le bouchon fait partie de la conception [Monsen and Baer 1992 - lots 89-93] trouvent une place toute naturelle dans la même vitrine que des flacons à bouchon en couronne. Rares sont ceux qui peuvent s'empêcher de sourire en contemplant un groupe de flacons à bouchon en couronne.

Die gekrönten Häupter des Parfüms

Dieser Artikel ist Pauline de Morcia gewidmet, die immer an ihrer Liebe zu Kronen-Stöpseln (im weiteren Artikel "crown-tops" genannt) und der am Sammeln teilhaben liess.

Der Gebrauch von Porzellanbehältern für Parfüm hat eine lange Geschichte. Erstaunliche frühe Beispiele wurden von den Meissen-Manufakturen im Deutschland des späten 18. Jahrhunderts und während der nächsten hundert Jahre produziert. Diese skulpturähnlichen Miniatur-Flakons enthalten oft ein humorvolles Überraschungselement. Ein ausgezeichnetes Beispiel dafür ist eine sehr alte Meissen Flasche in Form eines Mönchs, der eine Weizengarbe trägt (cf. Martin 1982, p. 13). Beim Abnehmen des Kopfstöpsels des Mönchs enthüllt sich, dass ein Mädchen in der Weizengarbe versteckt ist. "Crown-top" Parfümflaschen sind auf dieser langen Tradition humorvoller figürlicher Porzellanflaschen aufgebaut. Vom späten 19. Jahrhundert bis hin zu 1930 wurden figürliche "crown-top" Parfümflaschen von deutschen Fabriken hergestellt. Die hunderte, ja vielleicht sogar tausende in verschiedenen Ausführungen, machen das Sammeln von "crown-tops" zu einer spannenden Herausforderung für den Parfümflaschen-Liebhaber.

Die meisten "crown-tops" wurden leer verkauft, um des Käufers bevorzugten Wohlgeruch aufzunehmen, jedoch wurden gelegentlich auch Exemplare mit Etiketten und Verpackungen gefunden, die darauf hinweisen, dass "crown-tops" auch von kommerziellen Parfümfirmen gebraucht wurden, um die Vermarktung ihres Produkts zu steigern. Der typische Stöpsel, welcher diesen Flaschen ihren Namen gibt, ist wie eine Krone geformt. Der Stöpsel, mit einem passenden Korken, ist eine zweiteilige Konstruktion, welche es erlaubt, die Flasche mit einem halben Dreh zu öffnen und zu schliessen. Dieser Shaker-artige Stil ist der gebräuchlichste Typ eines Stöpsels, aber man findet auch andere Arten, wie z.B. massive Kronen und massive in Blumenform hergestellte Stöpsel mit passenden Korken. In einigen Fällen schraubt sich die ganze Krone ab und man findet einen winzigen Ausgiesser in dem Korkenverschluss vor. Das Band um den Korken ist oft mit Deutschland markiert oder hat ein dekoratives Muster. Gelegentlich ist auch der Name eines Unternehmens auf diesem Band moduliert.

Die überwiegende Anzahl von Parfümen mit "crown-tops" wurde in Deutschland und

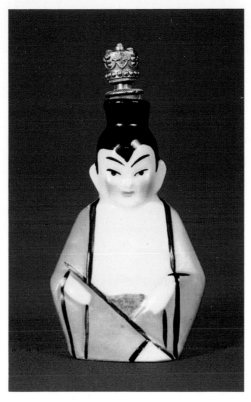

Figure 38. A Japanese figure in green robe; German manufacture.

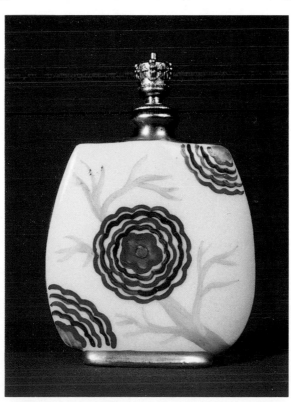

Figure 39. Hand-painted flask-type bottle, here decorated with stylized Art Deco flowers.

Bayern hergestellt. Andere Beispiele können aus Frankreich, Holland, Österreich, England und Japan gefunden werden. Die deutschen Exemplare sind in einer Vielzahl von Möglichkeiten markiert. Viele können mit einem auf dem Boden versehenen Tintenstempel gefunden werden, der Deutschland, Bayern, Made in Germany, oder manchmal sogar das Unternehmen zeigt, welches die Flasche importiert oder vertrieben hat. Diese Tintenstempel waren nicht immer unauslöschlich und sind deshalb manchmal sehr schwach oder sogar vollständig verschwunden. Es wurden auch eingeprägte Markierungen benutzt. Man findet oft Deutschland auf den Rücken oder auf die Seite der Flasche geprägt, auch sind sie oft mit einer Präge-Nummer verbunden. Diese eingeprägten Nummern scheinen Gussform-Nummern gewesen zu sein und sind manchmal das einzige Identifizierungs-Kennzeichen, das man auf der Flasche findet. Es existieren auch wunderschöne Exemplare mit überhaupt keinem Identifizierungs-Kennzeichen, die so zum Geheimnis des Sammelns beitragen.

Mehrere grosse Porzellan-Fabriken fertigten "crown-top" Flaschen an und benutzten zur Identifizierung ihr Firmenzeichen. Die Porzellan-Firmen Sitzendorf, Schneider, Schäfer & Vater und Goebel stellten alle "crown-top" Flaschen her. Die "crown-tops" des Goebel Unternehmens sind bei den Sammlern besonders populär. Sie sind besonders gut gekennzeichnet, einschliesslich umfassender Guss-Nummern und dem Kronen-Kennzeichen, welches zwischen 1935 und 1942 benutzt wurde. Die Qualität der Goebel Flaschen ist meistens ausserordentlich und von wunderschönem Humor und sorgfältigem Detail.

Der Sammler von "crown-tops" mag ein Generalist sein, der die breite Variante aller erhältlichen Formen sammelt, oder ein Spezialist, der sich auf eine spezifische Kategorie spezialisiert hat. Clowns und Pierrots, Orientalen, Ägypter und andere ethnische Figuren, Kinder und historische Damen sind einige der Kategorien, die den Sammler von menschlichen Figuren interessieren mag. Für den Tierfreund stellen "crown-tops" einen wahrhaften Zoo von Möglichkeiten dar, der Hunde, Katzen, Vögel, Insekten, Elefanten, Kamele, Bären und Löwen

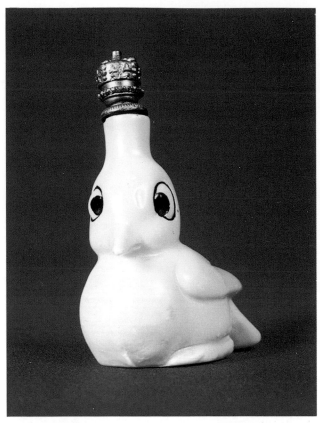

Figure 40. A Yellow Canary with big eyes.

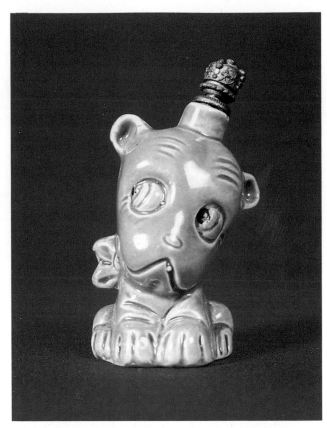

Figure 41. A brown Puppy, with huge paws and eyes.

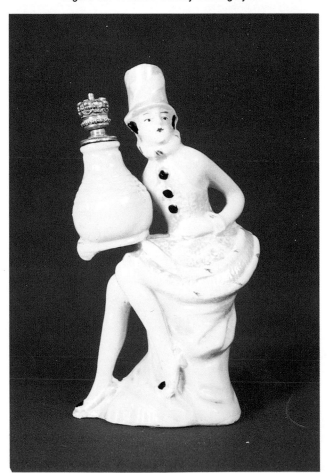

Figure 42. A woman dancer, holding a perfume urn.

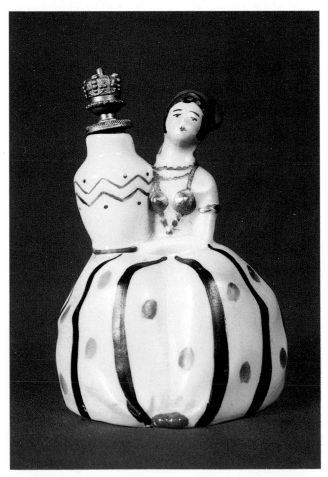

Figure 43. Woman in ball gown, holding a perfume urn.

beinhaltet. "Crown-tops" in der Form von Blumenkörben und Blumenvasen sind eine andere Möglichkeit. Art Deco Enthusiasten finden viele Beispiele in herrlichem Stil (Monsen & Baer 1995 - Lot #113). Eine kleine Gruppe von "crown-tops" ist wie Kewpie-Babies geformt. Ähnlich der Kewpie-Puppe die von Rose O'Neill in 1913 entworfen und patentiert wurde, jedoch ohne die blauen Flügel, gehören diese kleinen Flaschen zu den Favoriten unter den Sammlern. Unter den Kewpie-Flaschen sind fünf verschiedene Posen bekannt - Hände an den Beinen, Arme über dem Rücken verschränkt, Hände unter dem Kinn, Arme über der Brust gekreuzt und Arme entlang der Seite. Durch den subtilen Unterschied dieser Posen ist dieses Set schwierig zusammenzustellen und die Möglichkeit noch eine andere Pose zu finden, belebt das Abenteuer des Sammelns.

Ursprüglich als Novitäten verkauft, kosteten "crown-top" Parfüm-Flaschen wahrscheinlich nur ein paar Pennies. Die Wegwerf-Natur dieser Flaschen hat zu ihrer derzeitigen Rarität beigetragen. Der heutige Sammler muss mit einem Preis von etwas unter hundert Dollar für mehr alltägliche und bis zu mehreren hundert Dollar für sehr edle Exemplare rechnen. Wie mit allen Parfüm-Flaschen ist der Zustand von grosser Wichtigkeit. Sammler suchen nach Exemplaren von schöner Form, mit schön detaillierter Bemalung, ohne Schaden und mit der Krone. Während der "crown-top"-Stöpsel ein wesentlicher Bestandteil ist, sollte jedoch niemals jemand eine interessante Flasche ausschlagen, nur weil er fehlt.

Wie in allen Bereichen des Parfüm-Flaschen-Sammelns führt eine Kategorie zur anderen. Der Sammler von "crown-top" Porzellan-Flaschen mag sehr wohl bald auch an einigen der deutschen Glas-Flaschen Geschmack finden, die aus Mercury-Glas, oder aus milchweissem oder aus klarem Glas mit Farbwirbeln gemacht sind. Diese findet man gewöhnlich mit einem Mercury-Glasstöpsel, der wie ein Glasball mit einem Applikator geformt ist, aber dann und wann haben sie auch den typischen metallenen "crown-top"-Stöpsel. Ein anderer Typ einer Glas-Flasche mit einem "crown-top" ist das Gesicht mit weitaufgerissenen starren Augen, welches aus dünnem Milchglas gemacht ist (Monsen & Baer 1992 - Lot # 87). Figürliche Flaschen, bei denen der Stöpsel in den Entwurf einverleibt ist (Monsen & Baer 1992 - Lots #89-#93), sind auch natürliche "Gehäuse-Partner" mit "crown-tops". Es gibt wenige Leute, die ohne ein Lächeln über diese "Wohlgerüche von Humor" eine Gruppe von "crown-top"-Parfüme betrachten können.

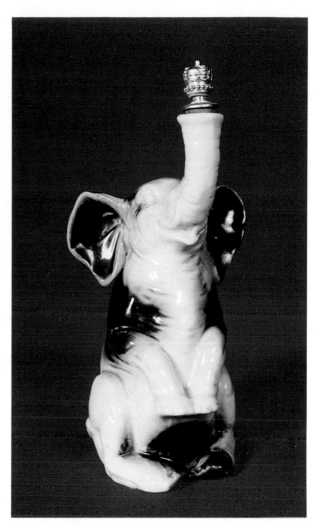

Figure 44. An elephant, with trunk up for good luck.

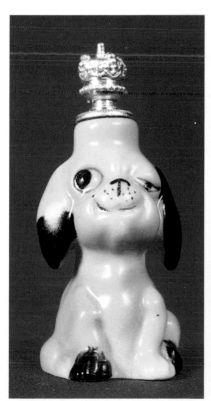

Figure 45. A cute dog, winking at us.

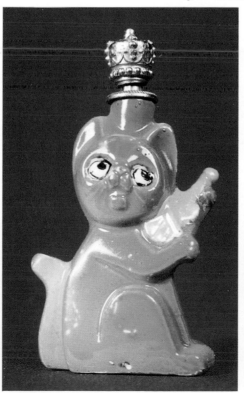

Figure 46. A green cat and yellow violin.

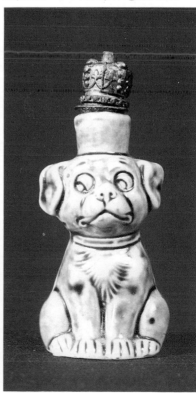

Figure 47. A happy little puppy.

CHRISTIAN DIOR
Symbol of French Elegance
Symbole de l'Elégance Française
Christie Mayer Lefkowith

Christian Dior was born on January 21, 1905, at Granville, France. His father was an industrialist and his mother a very elegant lady. To please his parents, he entered the School of Political Science to pursue a diplomatic career. Nevertheless he decided to abandon this path, and in 1928, barely 23 years old, he opened an art gallery with his friend Jacques Bonjean, the Gallery Jacques Bonjean. Having already numerous connections within the Parisian high society of the period — artists, art patrons, wealthy clients — he exhibited regularly (with great success) Chirico, Derain, Dufy, Léger, Maillol, Marcoussis, Matisse and occasionally Braque and Picasso. He also exhibited Christian Bérard and Jean Cocteau, who would become his close friends.

However, in 1931, he left Paris. Very upset by the recent death of his mother, he went to Russia for a study trip with a group of architects. Unfortunately, upon his return, he found his father ruined by the New York stock market crash. The financial crisis which ensued forced him to close the gallery, but he remained in the art world by joining the gallery of his friend, Pierre Colle. He exhibited there works by Salvador Dali, as he had a passion for the surrealist movement.

These activities in the art world would be short lived, since in 1934, gravely ill with tuberculosis, he had to leave for convalescence. Weakened and incapable of little else, he learned to make tapestry. In 1935, destitute, but obligated to help his family financially, he returned to Paris. A friend who took him in encouraged him to get into fashion design. Among his numerous first clients were the fashion designers Jean Patou, Nina Ricci, Marcel Rochas and Elsa Schiaparelli, the milliners Rose Valois and Suzy, and the newspaper Le Figaro. Obviously very talented,

Christian Dior naquit le 21 janvier 1905 à Granville, d'un père industriel, d'une mère très élégante. Pour satisfaire ses parents, il entra à l'Ecole des Sciences Politiques en vue d'une carrière diplomatique. Néanmoins il décida d'abandonner cette voie, et en 1928, à peine âgé de 23 ans, il ouvrit une galerie d'art avec son ami, Jacques Bonjean; la Galerie Jean Bonjean. Ayant déjà de nombreuses relations parmi le Tout-Paris de l'époque — artistes, mécènes, clients fortunés — il exposa régulièrement, et avec grand succès, Chirico, Derain, Dufy, Léger, Maillol, Marcoussis, Matisse et quelquefois Braque et Picasso. Il exposa également Christian Bérard et Jean Cocteau, qui allaient devenir ses amis proches.

Pourtant en 1931, il quitta Paris. Très touché par le récent décès de sa mère, il partit en Russie avec un groupe d'architectes pour un long voyage d'études. Malheureusement à son retour, il trouva son père ruiné par le krach boursier de New York. La crise financière qui en découla, l'obligea à fermer la galerie, mais il resta dans le domaine artistique en s'associant à la galerie de son ami, Pierre Colle. Passionné pour le surréalisme, c'est là qu'il exposa Salvador Dali.

Ces activités dans le monde des arts devaient être de courte durée, car en 1934, gravement atteint de tuberculose, il dut partir en convalescence. Affaibli, et ne pouvant pas faire grand-chose, il apprit à faire de la

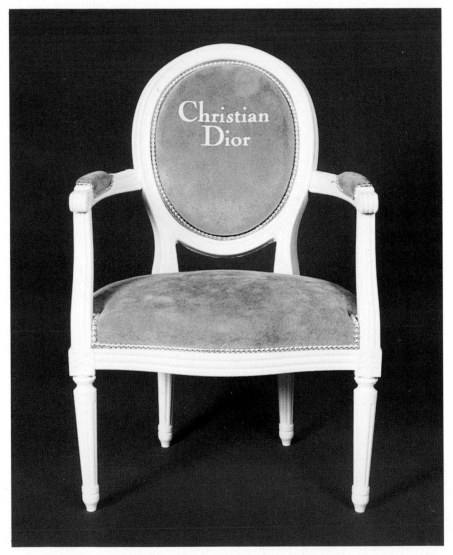

Figure 1. Christian Dior miniature display chair, symbol of the Dior style. Height: 11 3/4" [30 cm]. Collection of Christie and Ed Lefkowith.

tapisserie. En 1935, totalement démuni, et obligé d'aider financièrement sa famille, il revint à Paris. Un ami qui l'hébergeait, l'encouragea à se lancer dans le dessin de mode. Parmi ses nombreux premiers clients il y eut les couturiers, Jean Patou, Nina Ricci, Marcel Rochas et Elsa

he was counseled and encouraged by Michel de Brunhoff, then editor-in-chief of French *Vogue*. The following year his designs were bought by, among others, Cristobal Balenciaga, Edward Molyneux, Worth, Lilly Daché and the magazine *Vogue*.

From 1936 his life-style changed, and in 1937 he moved to a sumptuous apartment on Rue Royale. In 1938 he was hired as a designer at the couture house Robert Piguet. There, he designed three collections, and became famous for his *Café Anglais* dress, a forerunner model, and for his theater costumes. Drafted in 1939 and discharged in 1940, having lost his position at Piguet, he left to join his family at Caillan, near Grasse, where he continued to design for *Le Figaro*.

Upon his return to Paris in 1941, he was hired as a designer by Lucien Lelong. His personal style evolved then toward the *Belle Époque* style: constricted waist, flared skirts (especially toward the back), draped fabric. This was the style of his mother's youth, a mother whose elegance he had so admired. It was also the preferred style of movie actresses, hence the numerous costumes which he created for the great French films of the period.

As soon as the war had ended, the important textile industrialist, Marcel Boussac, proposed a permanent association to this creative genius. Thus supported by the powerful financial organization of Marcel Boussac, the company *Christian Dior S. A. R. L.* was established on October 8, 1946, at 30 Avenue Montaigne, in the magnificent 18th century building. The interior decor was executed by Victor Grandpierre following the very precise instructions of the great *couturier* himself, who wanted to create an atmosphere that was Parisian, classic, sober, and above all, elegant. The chosen style was the neo-Louis XVI style, carried out in gray and white only, with crystal and bronze lights and white lacquered furniture as the sole accessories. This style would be used in all the Christian Dior boutiques, in France as well as abroad, and would become the symbol of the Dior style. Thus, the little gray and white display chair [Fig. 1], in the Louis XVI style, would become the embodiment of the Dior style.

The 1947 Spring-Summer Collection was presented on February 12, 1947. On the program, two silhouettes were announced: "Corolla" (the outline of a flower) and "In 8." During and after the war, women dressed in an almost military fashion: a straight, short line, with square shoulders. But this new silhouette, typically feminine, was the opposite: small, rounded shoulders, emphasized bust, tightly corseted waist, round hips, and skirts that were either straight or full, but always at least at mid-calf length. "Your dresses have

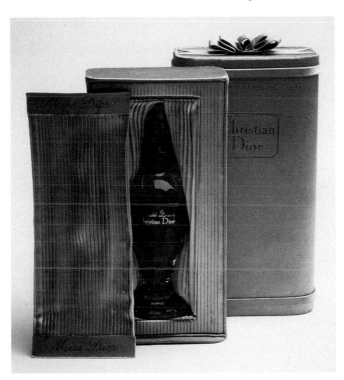

Figure 2. Christian Dior *Miss Dior*, 1947.
Collection of Christie and Ed Lefkowith.

Schiaparelli, les modistes Rose Valois et Suzy et le journal *Le Figaro*. Evidemment très doué, il fut conseillé et encouragé par Michel de Brunhoff, alors rédacteur en chef du V*ogue* Français. L'année suivante ses dessins furent achetés par, entre autres, Cristobal Balenciaga, Edward Molyneux, Worth, Lilly Daché et le magazine V*ogue*.

Dès 1936 son style de vie changea, et en 1937 il déménagea dans un sompteux appartement, rue Royale. En 1938 il entra comme modéliste dans la maison de couture Robert Piguet. Il y dessina trois collections et devint célèbre grace à la robe "Café anglais," un modèle précurseur, et à ses costumes conçus pour le théâtre. Mobilisé en 1939 et démobilisé en 1940, ayant perdu sa place chez Piguet, il partit joindre sa famille à Caillan, près de Grasse — où il continua à dessiner pour *Le Figaro*.

De retour à Paris en 1941, il fut engagé comme modéliste par Lucien Lelong. C'est là que son style personnel evolua vers le style "Belle Epoque": la taille creusée, les jupes évasées, surtout dans le dos, les drapés . C'était le style de la jeunesse de sa mère, cette mère dont il avait tant admiré l'élégance. C'était aussi le style préféré des actrices de cinema, d'où de nombreux costumes créés pour les grands films français de l'époque.

Dès la fin de la guerre, le grand industriel du textile, Marcel Boussac, proposa à ce créateur de génie une association permanente. C'est ainsi que soutenue par la puissante organisation financière de Marcel Boussac, la société Christian Dior S.A.R.L. fut constituée le 8 octobre 1946, au 30 avenue Montaigne, dans le magnifique immeuble XVIIIe. La décoration intérieure fut réalisée par Victor Grandpierre suivant les indications très précises du grand couturier lui-même, désireux de créer une atmosphère parisienne, classique, sobre et élégante. Le style choisi fut le style néo-Louis XVI, exécuté en gris et blanc uniquement, avec pour seuls accessoires le cristal et le bronze des luminaires et des meubles laqués en blanc. Ce style sera employé dans toutes les boutiques Christian Dior, aussi bien en France qu'à l'étranger, et deviendra le symbole du style Dior. Ainsi la petite chaise de vitrine (Figure 1) grise et blanche, de style Louis XVI, deviendra elle-même la concrétisation du style Dior.

La collection printemps-été 1947 fut présentée le 12 février 1947. Au programme, deux silhouettes furent annoncées: "corolle" et "en 8". Pendant et depuis la guerre les femmes s'habillaient en tenue presque militaire: de ligne droite, courte et à épaules carrées. Mais cette nouvelle silhouette, typiquement féminine, était à l'opposé: les épaules petites et arrondies, le buste souligné, la taille étranglée, les

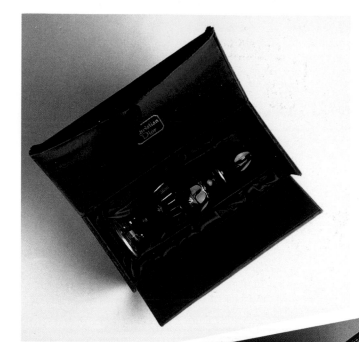

Figure 3. Christian Dior *Miss Dior*, 1947. Collection of Christie and Ed Lefkowith.

hanches rondes, les jupes soit droites, soit amples, mais toujours au moins à mi-mollet. "Your dresses have such a new look" dit à Christian Dior Carmel Snow, rédactrice en chef du *Harper's Bazaar*. Et ce fut "Le New Look", une révolution contre la libération du corps féminin, telle que l'avaient préconisée Paul Poiret et Coco Chanel.

Parmi les journalistes le succès fut énorme, ainsi que parmi les clientes parisiennes qui passèrent de nombreuses commandes. Mais les acheteurs des grands magasins américains étaient déjà repartis sans assister à la présentation de ce couturier dont ils n'avaient jamais entendu parler. Ils ont été donc obligés de revenir et passèrent, eux aussi, de nombreuses commandes. Marcel Boussac était ravi, car il fallait beaucoup de tissu pour exécuter cette nouvelle mode: jusqu'à 20 mètres pour une robe d'après-midi. Aussitôt les américaines se révoltèrent contre l'ampleur et la longueur des jupes — et contre la tyrannie de la mode parisienne. Un club fut immédiatement constitué: "The Little Below the Knee Club" ("Le Petit Club du Juste en Dessous du Genou").

Eventuellement "Le New Look" conquit les Etats-Unis, et en Septembre 1947, Monsieur Marcus, directeur d'un grand magasin de luxe américain, Nieman Marcus à Dallas, remit à Christian Dior, l'Oscar de la Couture. Cet immense succès américain contribua à l'ouverture d'une boutique, Christian Dior, New York, Inc., au coin de la 5`ème avenue et de la 57ème rue, et au lancement d'un premier parfum, *Miss Dior*, au nom américanisé.

Christian Dior, célèbre dans le monde

such a new look," Carmel Snow, editor of *Harper's Bazaar*, said to Christian Dior. Therefore, it was this "New Look" that served as a revolution against the liberation of the feminine body, a liberation which had been supported by Paul Poiret and Coco Chanel.

Success was overwhelming, not only among journalists, but also among the Parisian clients who placed numerous orders. But American department store buyers had already left Paris, without attending the fashion show of this designer who was un-

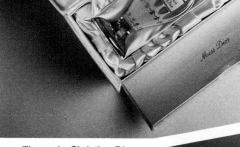

Figure 4. Christian Dior *Miss Dior*, 1947. Collection of Christie and Ed Lefkowith.

known to them. Therefore they had to return, so that they too could place numerous orders. Marcel Boussac was delighted, as a lot of fabric was required to produce these new fashions: up to 22 yards for just an afternoon dress. Immediately American women rebelled against the fullness and the length of the skirts—and against the tyranny of Parisian fashion. At once a club was formed: "The Little Below the Knee Club."

Eventually the "New Look" conquered the United States, and in September 1947, Mr. Marcus, head of the luxury department store Nieman Marcus in Dallas, presented Christian Dior with the Oscar of Couture. This extraordinary success in America contributed to the opening of a boutique, Christian Dior, New York, Inc., at the corner of 5th Avenue

Figure 5. [right] Christian Dior *Miss Dior*, 1947. Collection of Christie and Ed Lefkowith.

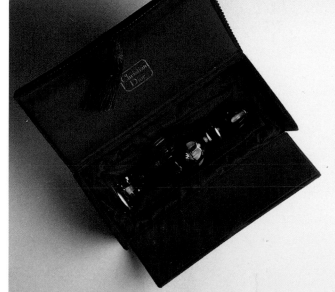

and 57th Street, and to the launch of a first perfume, *Miss Dior*, with its Americanized name.

Christian Dior, now famous world-wide, would establish a real empire—couture, furs, fashion accessories (such as hats, costume jewelry, purses, shoes, gloves, belts)—and especially perfumes—an empire which would outlive him. From then on, he would create two new collections each year, two new silhouettes, events which were eagerly awaited by the Press. Meanwhile he continued to create costumes for the great actresses of the period, such as Marlene Dietrich, Ava Gardner, Olivia de Havilland, Myrna Loy, and in 1954 he received an Oscar nomination for the costumes of the film: *Indiscretion of an American Wife*.

In 1955, concerned perhaps with the future of his couture house, he hired the young Yves Saint-Laurent, whose talent he had already noticed. At the height of his public recognition, he appeared on the cover of the March 4, 1957 *Time* magazine. Unfortunately, on October 24 of the same year, he died of a stroke. He was only 52 years old.

Miss Dior, the first perfume [Fig. 2], was presented in an elegant amphora-shaped bottle, in clear Baccarat crystal which expressed perfectly the curvaceous form of the feminine body, suddenly glamourized by the "New Look." Later, there was a sumptuous identical model, in clear crystal overlaid in either blue [Fig. 3], or white [Fig. 4], or red crystal [Fig. 5], the three colors of the French flag which became fashionable after the Liberation of France. These three amphora-shaped bottles, in their magnificent fabric *coffrets*, were in perfect harmony not only with the classic decor of the couture salons, but also with the Dior style in general.

In 1949 *Di-*

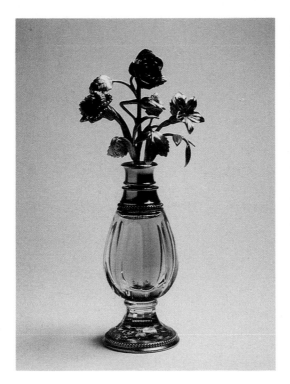

Figure 6. Christian Dior *Diorissimo*, 8.75" [22.3 cm]. Limited edition of 1956, bottle in clear crystal by Baccarat [#819]; the gilded bronze part designed and executed by Christiane Charles. Collection of Christie and Ed Lefkowith.

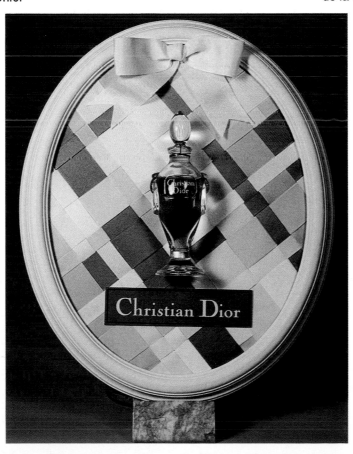

Figure 7. Christian Dior *Diorissimo*, 1956. Baccarat crystal bottle mounted on an oval display panel,16" [40.5 cm]. Collection of Christie and Ed Lefkowith.

entier allait établir un véritable empire — couture, fourrures, accessoires de mode, dont chapeaux, bijoux fantaisie, sacs, chaussures, gants, ceintures, etc. — et surtout parfums — un empire qui allait lui survivre. Dorénavant, il allait créer deux nouvelles collections par an, deux nouvelles silhouettes, événements toujours très attendus par la presse. Il continua cependant de créer des costumes pour les grandes actrices de l'époque, telles que Marlène Dietrich, Ava Gardner, Olivia de Havilland, Myrna Loy, et en 1954 il fut nominé aux Oscars du Cinéma pour les costumes du film: "Indiscretion of an American Wife" ("Indiscrétion d'une épouse américaine").

En 1955, soucieux peut-être de l'avenir de sa maison de couture, il engagea le jeune Yves Saint-Laurent dont il avait déjà remarqué le talent. Au comble de la reconnaissance publique, il parut en couverture du *Time* magazine, le 4 mars 1957. Malheureusement, le 24 octobre de la même année, il fut emporté par une attaque. Il avait à peine 52 ans.

Miss Dior, le premier parfum (Figure 2) fut présenté dans un élégant flacon en forme d'amphore, en cristal blanc de Baccarat, qui exprimait parfaitement les rondeurs du corps féminin, tout à coup mises en valeur par le "New Look". Plus tard, il y eut un somptueux modèle identique, en cristal doublé, soit de bleu (Figure 3), soit de blanc opaque (Figure 4), soit de rouge (Figure 5), les trois couleurs du drapeau tricolore mises à la mode par la libération. Les trois flacons-amphore, dans leur magnifiques écrins en tissu, s'harmonisaient parfaitement non seulement avec le décor classique des salons de la maison de couture, mais aussi avec le style Dior en général.

En 1949 *Di-*

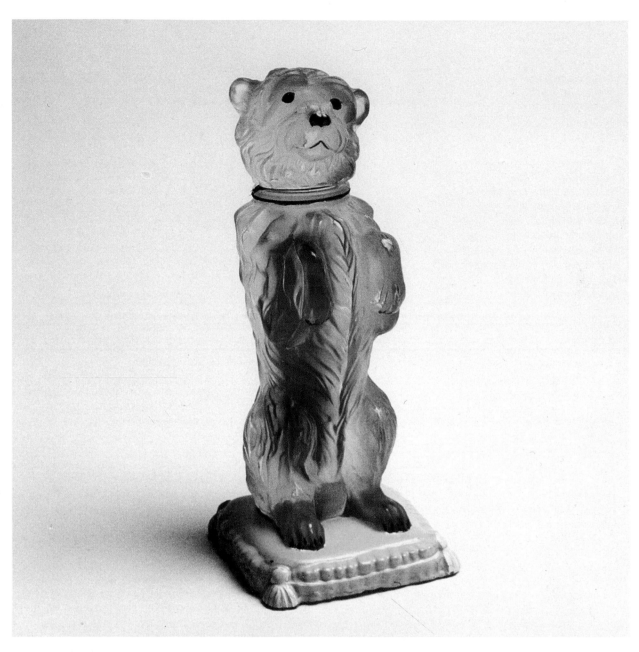

Figure 8. Christian Dior *J'appartiens à Miss Dior* ['I Belong to Miss Dior'], 1957, 7" [17.7 cm], limited edition. Collection of Christie and Ed Lefkowith.

orama was launched, also in an amphora-shaped bottle, and was named after the "Diorama" cocktail dress, in black wool, from the Fall/Winter collection of 1947—a Dior dress *par excellence*, since to make it 26 yards of extra-wide material were required, as well as 47 yards of braid, and 230 hours of work. The dress weighed almost seven pounds.

In 1956 *Diorissimo* was launched, a floral perfume with a base note of lily of the valley, the lucky flower of Christian Dior, who used it often to adorn many outfits in his collections. There even was a fashion line called "Muguet" ['lily of the valley'] in the Spring/Summer collection of 1954. The special edition of *Diorissimo* [Fig. 6] featured a superb bottle in clear Baccarat crystal amphora-shaped--or rather shaped like an inverted amphora—with its stopper crowned by a magnificent gilded bronze bouquet of flowers, conceived and executed by the great sculptor Chrystiane Charles. Its overall form strongly resembled the form of a crystal and gilded

orama fut lancé, également dans un flacon-amphore, et ainsi nommé d'après la robe d'après-midi habillée, en laine noire, *Diorama*, de la collection automne-hiver 1947 — la robe Dior par excellence, puisqu'il fallait pour la faire presque 24 mètres de tissu en grande largeur, 43 mètres de tresse, et 230 heures de travail. Elle pesait plus de 3 kilos.

En 1956 *Diorissimo* fut lancé, parfum floral à base de muguet, fleur fétiche de Christian Dior qui l'utilisait souvent en temps qu'ornement sur maintes toilettes de ses collections. Il y eut même une ligne "muguet", celle de la collection printemps-été 1954. L'édition spéciale de *Diorissimo* (Figure 6) comprenait un superbe flacon en cristal blanc de Baccarat en forme d'amphore — ou plutôt en forme d'amphore à l'envers — au bouchon coiffé d'un magnifique bouquet de fleurs en bronze doré, conçu et réalisé par le grand sculpteur Chrystiane Charles. Le tout ressemblait fort à un modèle de brûle-parfums en cristal et bronze doré

bronze Louis XVI perfume burner. Although metal had often been used previously in association with glass and crystal to create a feeling of luxury in perfume bottles, rarely, if ever, had a bronze sculpture of such singular beauty been created for this purpose. Perhaps even more remarkable was the fact that it was created in 1956, when superb design and workmanship were already becoming very scarce.

Miss Dior, *Diorama* and *Diorissimo* were exported worldwide, most often presented in a clear glass or crystal bottle, which was amphora-shaped and decorated with two symmetrical, fixed rings molded on each side of the bottle. Window displays of the period often included these amphora-shaped bottles, placed on oval shaped panels, lacquered white [Fig. 7]. These display panels were perfectly consistent with the interior and exterior oval mural decorations of the Christian Dior couture salons and boutiques. The white oval shape was also used as a graphic motif on the paper of various boxes for perfume bottles.

In 1957, to commemorate the 10th anniversary of the Dior house, of the "New Look" and of *Miss Dior*, a new presentation was created for *Miss Dior* [Fig. 8]—as an limited edition, possibly of only 350 examples. It was called *J'appartiens à Miss Dior* ['I Belong to Miss Dior']. The bottle, in the shape of a dog (Christian Dior's own bichon frisé) sitting up on a yellow enameled glass cushion, carried under its base a paper label numbered in Roman numerals and signed "Tian Dior" in the great couturier's own handwriting. Presented in an almost pagoda-shaped kennel, made of yellow silk with white trimmings, this little dog was offered only to selected clients and associates.

After the death of Christian Dior, Yves Saint-Laurent assumed the direction of the couture house. Branch stores and franchises multiplied. Other perfumes were created, as were many other beauty products—a sumptuous legacy, the continuation of the Dior style. This consistent style, which is found in all the Dior creations, has been wonderfully fixed in our memory by René Gruau's advertising images, symbols of the woman closely bound to her style and to her perfume [Figs. 9, 10, 11]. From the start, this friend of Christian Dior played a decisive role, because he was able to render the refined and luxurious feminine atmosphere which was inseparable not only from the Dior style, but also from the Dior era. Today other fashion designers and artists reinterpret the Christian Dior style, the eternal emissary of French elegance throughout the world.

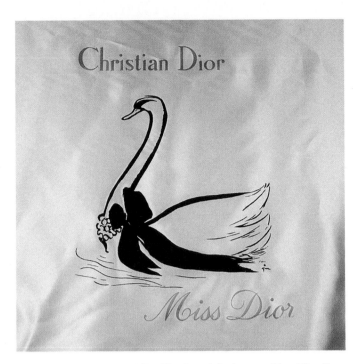

Figure 9. René Gruau *Miss Dior* signed display panel in white silk, 1947, 42" [107 cm]. Collection of Christie and Ed Lefkowith.

d'époque Louis XVI. Bien que déjà le métal ait souvent été utilisé en association avec le verre et le cristal, afin de donner aux flacons de parfum un aspect luxueux, rarement pour ne pas dire jamais, une sculpture en bronze d'une telle singulière beauté ne fut réalisée dans un tel but. Le plus extraordinaire est sans doute le fait que cette création date de 1956, époque à laquelle le génie de la création, et la qualité d'exécution étaient déjà devenus très rares.

Miss Dior, *Diorama* et *Diorissimo* ont été exportés dans le monde entier, le plus souvent présentés dans un flacon en verre ou en cristal blanc, en forme d'amphore, orné de deux anneaux fixes et symetriques, incorporés de chaque côté du flacon. La décoration des vitrines de l'époque comprenait souvent ces flacons en forme d'amphore, présentés sur des panneaux ovales, laqués blanc (Figure 7). Ces panneaux publicitaires s'assimilaient parfaitement aux formes ovales qui décoraient les murs intérieurs et extérieurs des salons de couture et des boutiques Christian Dior. L'ovale blanc était également utilisé en tant que motif graphique pour le papier de diverses boîtes à flacons de parfum.

En 1957, pour commémorer le 10ème anniversaire de la maison Dior, du "New Look" et de *Miss Dior*, une nouvelle présentation fut créée pour *Miss Dior* (Figure 8) — en édition limitée, possiblement à 350 exemplaires seulement. Elle s'appela *J'appartiens à Miss Dior*. Le flacon, en forme de chien (celui de Christian Dior), se dressant sur un coussin de verre laqué en jaune, portait sous la base une étiquette en papier numérotée en chiffres romains et signée "Tian Dior" de la main même du grand couturier. Présenté dans une boîte-niche presque en forme de pagode, en soie jaune soulignée de blanc, ce petit chien fut offert, seulement à certains clients et associés.

Après le décès de Christian Dior, Yves Saint-Laurent prit la direction de la maison de couture. Les succursales et les licences se multiplièrent. D'autres parfums furent créés, ainsi que maints produits de beauté — un héritage somptueux, la continuation du style Dior. Ce style cohérent, qui se retrouve dans toutes les créations Dior, a été merveilleusement fixé dans nos mémoires par les images publicitaires de René Gruau, symboles de la femme étroitement liée à son style et à son parfum (Figs. 9, 10, 11). Dès le départ, cet ami de Christian Dior joua un role décisif, car il sut recréer l'atmosphère féminine, raffinée et luxueuse, inséparable non seulement du style Dior, mais aussi de l'époque Dior. Aujourd'hui d'autres couturiers et artistes recréent le style Christian Dior, éternel emissaire de l'élégance française dans le monde entier.

Correspondence for the author can be addressed to:
Christie M. Lefkowith, FDR Station, PO Box 5200, New York, N.Y. 10150-5200.

CHRISTIAN DIOR - Symbol französischer Eleganz

Christian Dior wurde am 21. Januar 1905 in Granville, Frankreich, geboren. Sein Vater war Industrieller und seine Mutter eine sehr elegante Dame. Seinen Eltern zuliebe besuchte er die Schule für politische Wissenschaften bezüglich einer Diplomaten-Karriere, nichtsdestoweniger beschloss er jedoch diesen Pfad aufzugeben und eröffnete in 1928, gerade 23 Jahre alt, zusammen mit seinem Freund Jacques Bonjean eine Kunstgalerie: Die Galerie Jean Bonjean. Er hatte bereits mehrere Verbindungen zu der vornehmen Gesellschaft jener Zeit geknüpft - Künstler, Kunstmäzene, vermögende Klienten - und stellte mit grossem Erfolg regelmässig Chirico, Derain, Dufy, Léger, Maillol, Marcoussis, Matisse und manchmal Braque und Picasso aus, wie auch Christian Bérard und Jean Cocteau, die seine nahen Freunde werden sollten.

1931 verliess er jedoch Paris. Er war sehr bewegt über den vorangegangenen Tod seiner Mutter und begab sich mit einer Gruppe von Architekten auf eine Studienreise nach Russland. Bei seiner Rückkehr fand er unglücklicherweise seinen Vater durch den New Yorker Börsenkrach ruiniert vor. Die darauffolgende finanzielle Krise zwang ihn, die Gallerie zu schliessen, aber er blieb in der Welt der Kunst, indem er sich der Gallerie seines Freundes Pierre Colle anschloss. Er hatte eine Passion für den Surrealismus und stellte dort Salvador Dali aus.

Diese Aktivitäten in der Welt der Kunst waren jedoch von kurzer Dauer, da er sich in 1934, schwerkrank mit Tuberkulose, in Rekonvaleszenz begeben musste. Geschwächt und unfähig für etwas anderes, erlernte er Tapisserie. In 1935 kehrte er ohne Geldmittel, aber verpflichtet seiner Familie finanziell zu helfen, nach Paris zurück. Ein Freund nahm sich seiner an und ermutigte ihn zu Modeschöpfungen. Unter seinen zahlreichen ersten Kunden waren die Modeschöpfer Jean Patou, Nina Ricci, Marcel Rochas und Elsa Schiaparelli, die Modistinnen Rose Valois und Suzy und die Tageszeitung Le Figaro. Offensichtlich sehr talentiert, wurde er von Michel de Brunhoff, dem Chefeditor des französischen Vogue, beraten und ermutigt. Im folgenden Jahr wurden seine Entwürfe, unter anderen, von Christian Balenciaga, Edward Molyneux, Worth, Lilli Daché und dem Magazin Vogue gekauft.

Von 1936 an änderte sich sein Lebensstil und im Jahr 1937 zog er in ein prächtiges Appartement auf der Rue Royale. In 1938 begann er als Designer bei dem Couturier Robert Piguet. Er entwarf dort drei Kollektionen und wurde dank seines "Café Anglais"-Kleides, einem Vorläufer-Modell, und durch seine für das Theater entworfenen Kostüme berühmt. Er wurde in 1939 eingezogen und in 1940 entlassen. Da er seine Stelle bei Piguet verloren hatte, kehrte er zu seiner Familie nach Caillan, in der Nähe von Grasse, zurück und setzte fort für Le Figaro zu entwerfen.

Nach seiner Rückkehr nach Paris in 1941 wurde er als De-signer bei Lucien Lelong angestellt. Dort war es, dass sich sein persönlicher Stil in die Richtung des Belle Époque Stils entwickelte: Schmale Taille, bauschende Röcke, besonders im Rücken drapiertes Material. Dies war der Stil der Jugend seiner Mutter, deren Eleganz er so sehr bewunderte. Es war auch der bevorzugte Stil der Filmschauspielerinnen und demzufolge die grosse Anzahl der für den französischen Film dieser Zeit entworfenen Kostüme.

Sowie der Krieg vorüber war, bot der grosse Industrielle, Marcel Boussac, diesem kreativen Genie eine permanente Verbindung mit an. Unterstützt durch die mächtige Finanzorganisation von Marcel Boussac, wurde das Unternehmen Christian Dior S.A.R.L. am 8. Oktober 1946 in einem wunderschönen Gebäude des 18. Jahrhunderts in der Avenue Montaigne No. 30 eingerichtet. Die Innenausstattung wurde von Victor Grandpierre ausgeführt, indem er den sehr präzisen Angaben des grossen Modeschöpfers selbst folgte, der eine pariserische Atmosphäre schaffen wollte; Klassisch, nüchtern und vor allem - elegant. Der ausgewählte Stil war der des frühen Louis XVI, nur in weiss und grau ausgeführt, mit Kristall - und Bronzelampen und lackierten weissen Möbeln als einzigen Accessoires. Dieser Stil wurde in allen Christian Dior Boutiquen benutzt, sowohl in Frankreich als auch überall sonst, und wurde zum Symbol des Dior Stils. Auf diese Weise wurde der kleine weiss-graue Stuhl für das Schaufenster (Fig. 1), im Stil Louis XVI, zum konkreten Beispiel des Dior Stils.

Die Frühjahrs/ Sommer-Kollektion des Jahres 1947 wurde am 2. Februar 1947 präsentiert. Auf dem Programm waren zwei Silhouetten angekündigt: "Corolla" (der Umriss einer Blume) und "In 8". Während und auch nach dem Krieg waren Frauen fast in militärischer Manier gekleidet. Mit einer geraden, kurzen Linie und breitschulterig. Aber diese neue, typisch feminine Silhouette war gerade das Gegenteil. Kleine, gerundete Schultern, die Brust betont, die Taille eng geschnürt, runde Hüften, Röcke entweder gerade oder voll, aber immer mindestens halblang. "Ihre Kleider haben solch ein neues Aussehen", sagte Carmel Snow, Editor von Harper's Bazaar zu Christian Dior; und es war dieser "New Look", eine Revolution in Richtung auf die Befreiung des weiblichen Körpers, der von Paul Poiret und Coco Chanel befürwortet wurde.

Unter den Journalisten, wie auch unter der Pariser Kundschaft, die zahlreiche Bestellungen in Auftrag gab, war der Erfolg enorm. Jedoch waren die Einkäufer der grossen amerikanischen Warenhäuser schon abgereist, ohne der Präsentation dieses Modeschöpfers beizuwohnen, von dem sie noch nie gehört hatten. Also mussten sie zurückkommen und erteilten ebenfalls zahlreiche Aufträge. Marcel Boussac

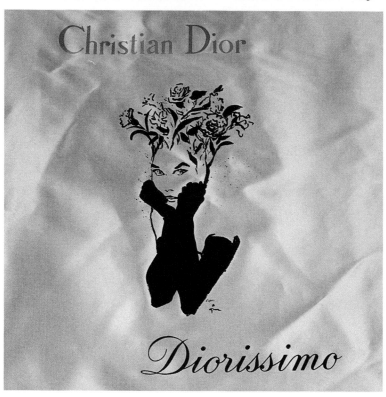

Figure 10. René Gruau *Diorissimo,* signed display panel in pink silk, 42" [107 cm], 1956. Collection of Christie and Ed Lefkowith.

war hoch erfreut, da es eine Menge an Material bedurfte, diese neue Mode herzustellen: Bis zu 20 Meter für lediglich ein Tageskleid. Die Amerikaner begannen bald gegen die Fülle und die Länge der Röcke zu revoltieren, wie auch gegen die Tyrannei der Pariser Mode. Es wurde sofort eine Vereinigung mit den Namen "Der unter dem Knie Club" gegründet.

Letztendlich besiegte der "New Look" die Vereinigten Staaten und Mr. Marcus, Chef des Luxus-Warenhauses Nieman Marcus in Dallas, Texas, sandte Christian Dior im September 1947 den Oscar der Couture. Dieser immense Erfolg in Amerika trug dazu bei, dass eine Boutique Christian Dior, New York, Inc. an der Ecke der 5. Avenue und der 57. Strasse eröffnet wurde und um den Start eines neuen Parfüms mit dem amerikanisierten Namen *Miss Dior* zu feiern.

Christian Dior wurde in der ganzen Welt berühmt und gründete ein wahrhaftiges Mode-Empire; Pelze, Mode-Accessoires wie Hüte, Modeschmuck, Taschen, Schuhe, Handschuhe, Gürtel und besonders Parfüme. Ein Reich, welches ihn selbst überleben sollte. Von nun an entwarf er jedes Jahr zwei Kollektionen, zwei neue Erscheinungsformen, und diese Ereignisse wurden von der Presse ungeduldig erwartet. Trotzdem kreierte er weiterhin Kostüme für die grossen Darstellerinnen dieser Zeit, wie Marlene Dietrich, Ava Gardner, Olivia de Havilland, Myrna Loy und wurde in 1954 aufgrund seiner Kostümentwürfe für den Film "Indiscretion of an American Wife" (Indiskretion einer amerikanischen Frau) für einen Oscar nominiert.

In 1955, in Achtsamkeit auf die Zukunft seines Mode-Unternehmens, stellte er den jungen Yves Saint-Laurent ein, auf dessen Talent er bereits aufmerksam geworden war. Auf der Höhe seines öffentlichen Ruhms wurde Christian Dior auf dem Titel des TIME - Magazins vom 4. März 1957 abgebildet. Bedauerlicherweise starb er am 24. Oktober des gleichen Jahres. Er wurde nur 52 Jahre alt.

Das erste Parfüm *Miss Dior* (Fig. 2) wurde in einer eleganten Flasche in Form einer Amphora aus klarem Kristall von Baccarat präsentiert und drückte perfekt die gerundete Form des weiblichen Körpers aus, die so plötzlich durch den "New Look" modern geworden war.

Später gab es ein prachtvolles identisches Modell in farbigem Kristallschliff: Blau (Fig. 3), weiss (Fig. 4) oder rot (Fig. 5), den drei Farben der französischen Flagge, modisch wiedergegeben aufgrund der Befreiung Frankreichs. Diese drei Amphora-Flaschen, in ihren prächtigen mit Tuch ausgeschlagenen Schachteln, befinden sich in vollkommener Eintracht nicht nur mit dem klassischen Dekor der Räume der "Maison de Couture", sondern auch mit dem Dior-Stil selbsthin.

In 1949 wurde *Diorama* vorgestellt, ebenfalls in einer Amphora-Flasche und nach dem nachmittäglichen Cocktail-Kleid aus schwarzer Wolle *Diorama* der Herbst/Winter-Kollektion des Jahres 1947 benannt - ein Dior-Kleid in höchster Vollendung, da 24 Meter von extra breitem Material, 43 Meter an Verzierungen und 230 Stunden Arbeitszeit zur Herstellung benötigt wurden. Das Kleid wog mehr als 7 Kilo.

Diorissimo wurde in 1956 herausgebracht, ein florales Parfüm auf Maiglöckchen-Basis, eine für Dior sinnbildliche Blume,

die er oft als Dekoration auf vielen Accessoires seiner Kollektion benutzte. Es gab sogar einen Modestil "Muguet" (Maiglöckchen) in der Frühjahrs/Sommer-Kollektion des Jahres 1954. Die Sonderausgabe von *Diorissimo* (Fig. 6) beinhaltete eine herrliche Flasche aus klarem Kristall von Baccarat in der Form einer Amphora - oder Moreso, einer umgedrehten Amphora - mit einem Stöpsel, der mit einem grossartigen goldbronzenen Blumenstrauss gekrönt war, erdacht und ausgeführt von der grossen Bildhauerin Chrystiane Charles.

Das ganze ähnelte sehr stark der Form einer Parfüm-Lampe in Kristall und Goldbronze aus der Zeit Louis XVI. Obwohl Metall oft in Verbindung mit Glas und Kristall verwandt wurde, um den Parfümflaschen eine luxuriöse Qualität zu verleihen, wurde jedoch selten oder sogar nie eine Skulptur von solch einzigartiger Schönheit für solch eine Verbindung benutzt. Das Ausserordentlichste daran ist, dass diese Kreation auf das Jahr 1956 zurückdatiert, einer Zeit, in welcher kreative Begabung und qualitative Ausführung bereits sehr selten waren.

Miss Dior, *Diorama* und *Diorissimo* wurden in die ganze Welt exportiert, meistens in einer Flasche aus klarem Glas oder Kristall, in der Form einer Amphora, dekoriert mit zwei symmetrischen auf jeder Seite der Flasche befestigten Ringen. Sehr oft waren die Schachteln dieser Flaschen in einer ovalen Form dekoriert, einer Form, die oft für viele Reklamezwecke benutzt wurde (Fig. 7). Diese ovale Form erinnert an die klassischen ovalen Paneele der Louis XVI Ära, mit welchen die Aussen- und Innenwände der Christian Dior Boutiquen dekoriert waren. In 1957, zum Gedenken des 10-jährigen Bestehens des Hauses Dior sowie des "New Look" und von *Miss Dior*, wurde eine neue Kreation für *Miss Dior* geschaffen (Fig. 8), und zwar in einer Ausgabe von möglicherweise nur 350 Exemplaren. Sie wurde *J'appartiens à Miss Dior* (Ich gehöre Miss Dior) genannt. Die Flasche, in der Form eines Hundes (Christian Dior's eigenem Bichon Frisé) der auf einem emaillierten gelben Kissen sitzt, trug auf der Unterseite ein Papieretikett mit römischen Ziffern und war in des grossen Modeschöpfers eigener Handschrift mit "Tian Dior" signiert. Dieser kleine Hund, in seiner fast einer Pagode ähnelnden Hunderhütte, die mit gelber Seide und weiss getrimmt ausgeschlagen war, wurde nur bestimmten Kunden und Geschäftsfreunden dargeboten.

Nach dem Tode Christian Dior's übernahm Yves Saint-Laurent die Direktion des Couture-Hauses. Es entstanden zahlreiche Zweigstellen und Konzessionen, andere Parfüme wurden geschaffen wie auch viele andere Schönheitsprodukte — eine kostbare Erbschaft, die Weiterführung des Dior Stils. Dieser kohärente Stil, in allen Dior Kreationen zu finden, ist durch René Gruau's Reklameabbildungen, Sinnbilder von Frauen, die eng an Mode und Parfüm gebunden sind (Fig. 9, 10 und 11), wunderbar in unserer Erinnerung befestigt. Dieser Freund Christian Dior's spielte von Beginn an eine ausschlaggebende Rolle, da er befähigt war, die verfeinerte und luxuriöse feminine Atmosphäre zu schaffen, welche nicht nur vom Dior Stil, sondern auch von dem dieser ganzen Ära untrennbar war. Andere Designer und Künstler geben heutzutage in der ganzen Welt den Stil Dior's wieder, des ewigen Emissärs französischer Eleganz.

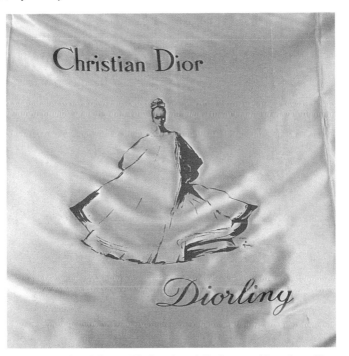

Figure 11. René Gruau *Diorling* signed display panel in yellow silk, 42" [107 cm], 1963. Collection of Christie and Ed Lefkowith.

ROBJ

Perfume Lamps, Powder Jars, Perfume — Brûle-parfums, Poudriers, et Parfums

Randall B. Monsen

The name *Robj* is associated with French decorative arts of the highest quality in both design and execution, yet very little is known today about the company that produced these beautiful objects. The name of the company derives from the name of its founder, Jean Born, since *Robj* is a spelling of some of the letters of his name arranged in reverse [n**roB** nae**J**]. The result is as difficult to pronounce in French as it is in English, but most people tend to say [robzh]. Jean Born evidently founded the company in 1908; by 1910 he was particularly intrigued by the use of electric lights in decorative lighting, and in that year he registered several models as *brûle-parfums*, or 'perfume burners.' The activities of the company are difficult to trace from its founding until the mid-nineteen twenties, when it was actively producing some of the most sublime creations of what we now call the "Art Deco Era." Lucien Willemetz was a major stockholder of the *Societé Jean Born & Cie.*, and in fact he took over the company when its founder was suddenly killed in a car accident in 1928. Willemetz had strong connections with the world of the theatre and the arts; his brother was the famous composer and lyricist of Mistinguett and Maurice Chevalier. He even exhibited *Robj* creations in the theaters of the time.

Robj commissioned work from some of the finest French artists and designers of the 1920's, and a collection of *Robj* is therefore a tapestry of French artistic talent from the Art Deco era. *Robj* actually sponsored artistic contests with monetary prizes among French artists of the era. Among the designers of *Robj* are the following: Edouard Martin, Raoul Mabru, Pierre Toulgonat, Jean Courtebassis, Henri Martin, Jeanne Lavergne, Marthe Coulon, and Georges Laurent. What makes *Robj* objects different from many other types of decorative art is that they embody the rarest of all attributes of art: a sense of humor and charm. *Robj* objects are never ponderous, depressingly serious, or grim, and because of this their high artistic quality is overlooked by some. *Robj* objects can seduce the viewer with their clear exemplification of the Art

Le nom Robj est associé aux arts décoratifs français de la plus haute qualité, tant dans leur exécution que dans leur conception, et pourtant cette société qui a produit ces beaux objets est largement inconnue. Le nom de la société est formé d'après le nom de son fondateur, Jean Born, puisque *Robj* est un anagramme de son nom écrit à l'envers [n**roB** nae**J**]. Le nom est difficile: on le prononce généralement [robzh]. Jean Born a apparemment fondé la société en 1908; déjà en 1910 il était intrigué par l'utilisation des lampes électriques dans l'éclairage décoratif; cette année-là il déposa plusieurs modèles de brûle-parfums. Les activités de la société sont difficiles à déterminer avant les années 20, date à laquelle elle produisait activement beaucoup des plus sublimes créations de ce que nous appelons maintenant l'époque Art Déco. Lucien Willemetz était un actionnaire important de la *Société Jean Born & Cie.*; d'ailleurs il la prit en main lors du décès inopiné du fondateur dans un accident d'automobile en 1928. Willemetz avait de nombreux liens avec le monde du théâtre et des arts; son frère était le célèbre compositeur et parolier de Mistinguett et de Maurice Chevalier. Il exposa même des créations *Robj* dans les théâtres de l'époque.

Robj passa des commandes aux meilleurs artistes des années 20; d'où le fait qu'une collection *Robj* est une fresque des talents français de l'époque Art Déco. *Robj* alla jusqu'à lancer des concours artistiques couronnés de récompenses monétaires. Parmi les artistes français ayant travaillé pour *Robj* on peut compter Edouard Martin, Raoul Mabru, Pierre Toulgonat, Jean Courtebassis, Henri Martin, Jeanne Lavergne, Marthe Coulon et Georges Laurent. Ce qui différencie les objets *Robj* de beaucoup d'autres types d'arts décoratifs est qu'ils incarnent l'attribut artistique le plus rare: le sens de l'humour et du charme. Les objets *Robj* ne sont jamais pondéreux, maussades ou d'un sérieux déprimant, ce qui empêche certains de percevoir leur beauté. Les objets *Robj* séduisent l'amateur par leur caractère nettement Art Déco, par leur capacité ingénieuse de pourvoir à un besoin

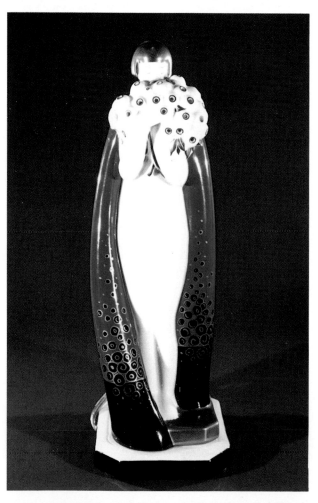

Figure 1. A statuesque Robj perfume lamp, two pieces, in the shape of an elegant nude; the perfume escapes through holes in her bouquet.

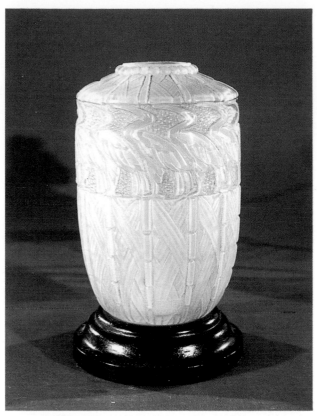

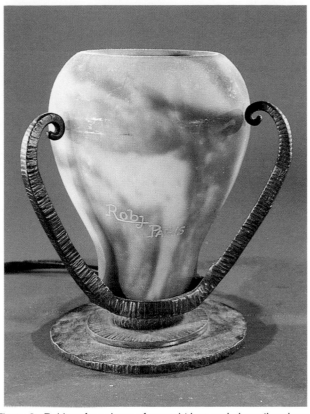

Figure 2. Robj glass perfume lamp molded with a row of exotic birds; the well for the perfume is an indention on top.

Figure 3. Robj perfume lamp of wrought iron and glass; the glass shade occurs in several different colors.

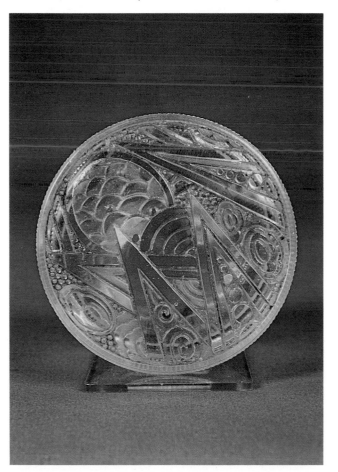

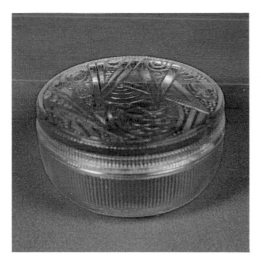

Figure 4-5. Robj glass dresser box, with a beautiful Art Deco design molded into the cover.
Collection of Randall B. Monsen and Rodney L. Baer.

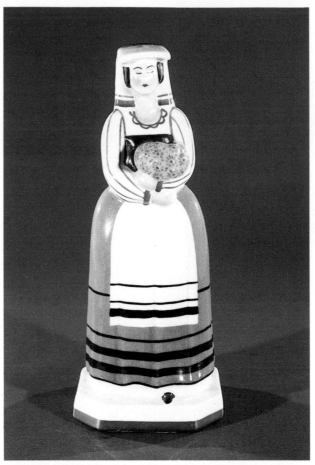

Figure 6. Robj porcelain perfume lamp molded in one piece.

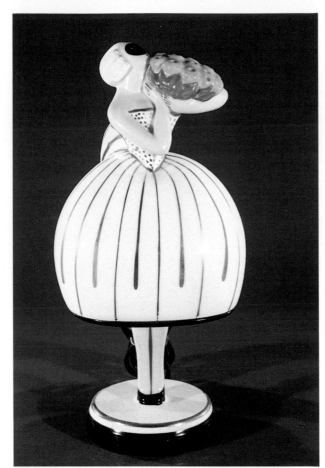

Figure 7. Robj porcelain perfume lamp, two pieces.

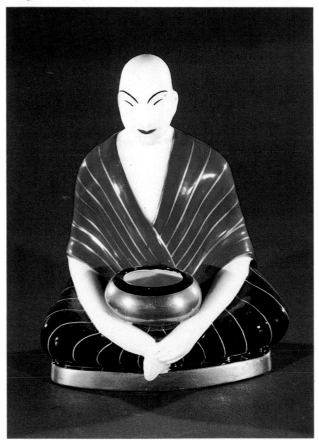

Figure 8. Robj perfume lamp in the shape of an Oriental man.

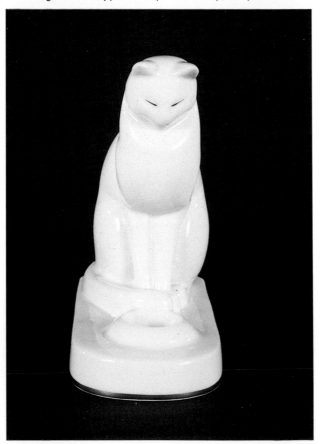

Figure 9. Robj porcelain perfume lamp; perfume is the cat's milk.

Deco style, by their ingenious ability to serve a mundane household function, but most often, merely by their charming whimsicality.

The Paris gallery where *Robj* was retailed was described in *Art et Décoration* in February 1929. The store was designed by the architect and designer René Herbst. According to this report of Herbst's design, his goal was unique. "*Robj* decorative objects are of two types: ornamental or functional ceramic objects on the one hand and lighting fixtures [lamps, night-lights, perfume burners] on the other hand. It was important therefore to adopt two different parts to the gallery, to throw light upon the first type and to underscore the light-giving capacity of the second type, without at the same time breaking the unity of the ensemble." The company used the following motto, which is no less true today: "Les bibelots *Robj* sont le complément de tout intérieur élégant," or "The bibelots of *Robj* complement every elegant interior decor."

Robj did produce decorative figurines solely to beautify the interior decor, but more commonly, *Robj* objects satisfy a common function in addition. Often a whimsical and transparent connection exists between the function of the object and its design. For example, there is a perfume lamp in the form of a monk holding a censer, and several others which depict women holding bouquets of flowers. The object "tells" the viewer its function. *Robj* objects include all of the following: liquor bottles, inkwells, powder jars, *bonbonières*, ashtrays, soap trays, *vide-poches*, bookends,

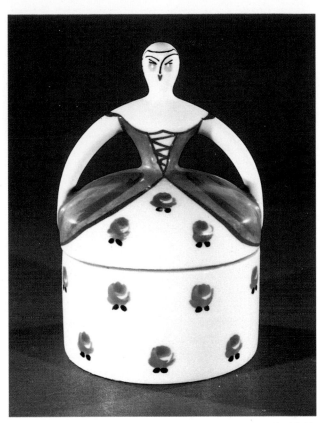

Figure 10. Robj porcelain powder jar in the shape of a highly stylized Art Deco lady, this model occurs in several colors.

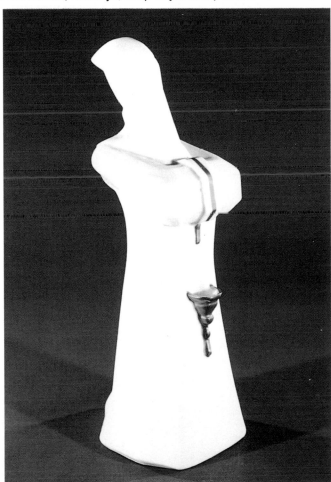

Figure 11. Robj white porcelain perfume lamp [one piece]; a hooded monk carrying--appropriately--an incense burner.

quotidien, mais le plus souvent par leur charme fantaisiste.

La galerie parisienne de *Robj* est décrite dans le numéro de février d'*Art et Décoration*. La boutique était l'oeuvre de l'architecte René Herbst. Selon cette description de la conception de Herbst il avait un but unique. "Ces bibelots sont de deux sortes: céramiques ornementales ou d'usage d'une part, objets lumineux d'autre part (lampes, veilleuses, brûle-parfums). Il importait par conséquent d'adopter deux partis différents, pour éclairer les premières et pour faire ressortir les qualités éclairantes des seconds, sans rompre toutefois l'unité de l'ensemble." La société affichait la devise suivante: "Les bibelots Robj sont le complément de tout intérieur élégant."

Même si *Robj* produisit des figurines décoratives dont la seule justification était leur beauté, le plus souvent les objets *Robj* ont une utilité quotidienne. Il y a souvent un lien fantaisiste entre la fonction de l'objet et son dessin. Par exemple, il y a un brûle-parfum en forme de moine tenant un encensoir, et d'autres de femmes tenant des bouquets de fleurs. L'objet 'affiche' sa fonction à l'utilisateur. Parmi les objets *Robj* on trouve des flacons à spiritueux, des encriers, des poudriers, des bonbonières, des cendriers, des porte-savons, des vide-poches, des serres-livres, des brûle-parfums, des cocktail shakers, des pots de crème, des pots de confiture, des lampes, des cloches à pain et à fromage, des théières et des cafetières, des biscuitières, des tabatières, des tasses et soucoupes, des sucriers, des pots à lait, des pieds de verres à liqueur, des horloges, des porte-thermomètres, des presse-oranges, des masques

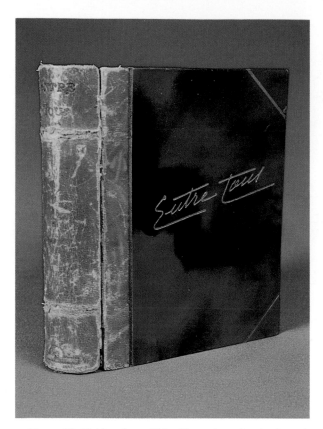

Figure 12. Robj perfume *Entre Tous*, whose box is shaped exactly like a leather bound book.
Collection of Randall B. Monsen and Rodney L. Baer.

perfume lamps, cocktail shakers, cream pots, jam pots, lamps, cake and cheese bells, tea and coffee pots, cookie jars, tobacco jars, cups and saucers, sugar bowls, milk pitchers, liquor glass holders, clocks, thermometer holders, orange reamers, wall masks, and many other things. The liquor bottles were very popular in the United States, possibly because the [tongue-in-cheek] concealment of liquor was a necessary part of the Prohibition era. *Robj* also produced art glass in brilliant colors, as well as a line of commercial perfume [*Le Sécret du Robj* and *Entre Tous*], and a great variety of lighting fixtures made of bronze and art glass.

Robj made a great variety of powder jars of all sizes, some even large enough to conceal a small bottle of whiskey. They are typically in the form of a woman in a very full skirt, and many different designs were used. Porcelain was ideally suited to the creation of perfume lamps, since it is highly translucent when illuminated from within. The heat of the light would make the perfume rapidly diffuse into the surrounding air. Some perfume lamps were also made of very fine art glass on a bronze or wood base. The glass in this case is of very fine quality, and would be made with an indented well for the perfume at the top. By the close of the twentieth century, the custom of burning perfume has fallen into disuse. However, the idea of burning perfume, or of heating it to diffuse it, dates from the very origin of perfume, whose name literally means 'through the smoke.' None of the Robj perfumes appears to have been a great commercial success, and all should probably be considered relatively rare. In some cases, circa 1928, *Robj* perfumes [whose exact names would be interesting to know] were bottled in crystal made by Baccarat, with stoppers in the shape of crowns.

muraux, et bien d'autres choses. Les flacons à spiritueux étaient très recherchés aux USA, car la Prohibition (l'interdiction de vente d'alcools de 1919 à 1933) rendait nécessaire le déguisement de tout contenant d'alcool. *Robj* fit également du verre artistique dans des couleurs brillantes ainsi qu'une gamme commerciale de parfums [*Le Secret du Robj* et *Entre Tous*], et une grande variété de lampes faites de bronze et de verre d'art.

Robj produisit un grand nombre de poudriers, dont certains capables de cacher une petite bouteille de whiskey. Le plus souvent elles ont la forme d'une femme avec une grande jupe et elles connurent de nombreuses formes. La porcelaine était le matériel idéal pour les brûle-parfums puisque la porcelaine éclairée à l'intérieur est translucide. La chaleur de la lumière diffusait rapidement le parfum dans l'air environnant. Certains brûle-parfums étaient en verre d'art fin sur un socle en bronze ou en bois. Le verre dans ce cas était d'une grande qualité avec un réceptacle en haut pour le parfum. A la fin du vingtième siècle, la pratique de brûler le parfum est tombée en désuétude. Mais la notion de brûler le parfum, ou de le chauffer pour le diffuser remonte à l'origine même du parfum, qui veut dire litéralement "par la fumée". Aucun des parfums de *Robj* ne semble avoir été un grand succès commercial et ils devraient probablement être considérés comme relativement rares. Dans certains cas, vers 1928, des parfums *Robj* [dont il serait intéressant de connaître les noms exacts] étaient vendus dans des flacons de cristal de Baccarat, avec des bouchons en forme de couronne.

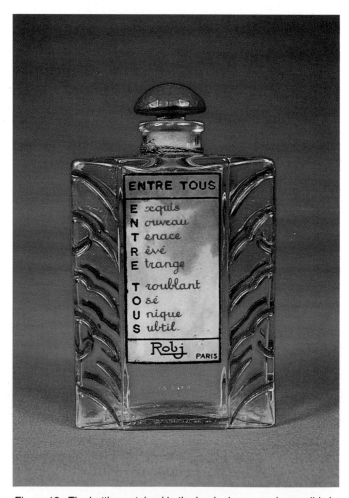

Figure 13. The bottle contained in the book above, made possibly by one of the early French glass artists, such as Dépinoix.

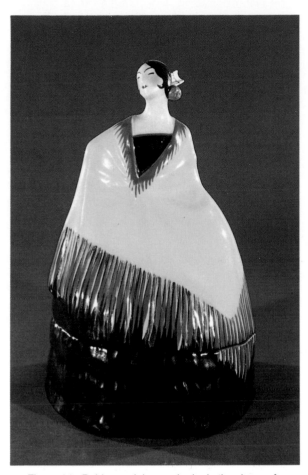

Figure 14. Robj porcelain powder jar in the shape of a Spanish lady with a bright shawl; this model is found painted with numerous different colors.

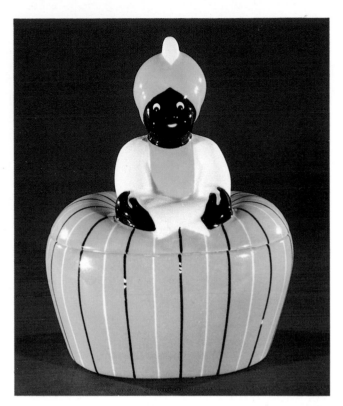

Figure 15. Robj powder jar in the shape of a turbaned black man.

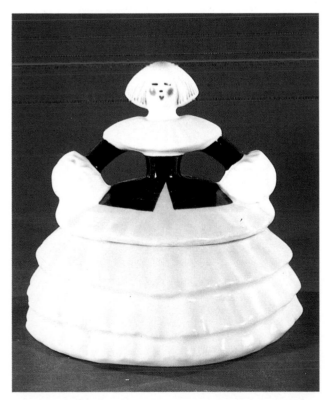

Figure 16. Robj powder jar in the shape of a lady in Art Deco style.

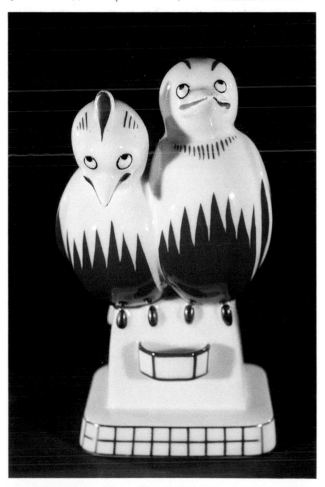

Figure 17. Robj porcelain perfume lamp with two lovebirds, showing the ability of Robj objects to combine both elegance and humor.

ROBJ - Parfüm-Lampen, Puderdosen, Parfüme

Der Name Robj ist mit der französischen dekorativen Kunst von höchster Qualität verbunden, sowohl im Entwurf als auch in der Ausführung, jedoch ist bis heute sehr wenig über das Unternehmen selbst bekannt, welches diese schönen Objekte produzierte. Der Name des Unternehmens wurde aus dem Namen seines Gründers hergeleitet, Jean Born; denn Robj ist eine Zusammenstellung einiger Buchstaben seines Namens in umgekehrter Reihenfolge (nROB naeJ). Das Ergebnis ist in französisch genauso schwer auszusprechen wie in englisch, jedoch tendieren die meisten Leute (robzh) zu sagen. Jean Born hat die Firma offensichtlich in 1908 gegründet; bis 1910 war er insbesondere von dem Gebrauch elektrischen Lichts in der dekorativen Beleuchtung fasziniert und liess in diesem Jahr mehrere Modelle als "brûle-parfums" oder "Parfüm-Lampen" eintragen. Die Aktivitäten des Unternehmens sind von seiner Gründung bis zur Mitte der 20-er Jahre schwer erforschbar, in welchen es einige der hochgradigsten Kreationen schuf, die wir heute die "Art-Deco-Epoche" nennen. Lucien Willemetz war einer der Hauptaktionäre der "Societé Jean Born & Cie." und übernahm in der Tat das Unternehmen als sein Gründer in 1928 aufgrund eines Autounfalls plötzlich getötet wurde. Willemetz hatte sehr enge Kontakte zu der Welt des Theaters und der Kunst; sein Bruder war der berühmte Komponist und Textdichter der Mistinguett und Maurice Chevalier's. Er stellte sogar Robj-Kreationen in den Theatern dieser Zeit aus.

Robj beauftragte einige der besten französischen Künstler und Designer mit Arbeiten und eine Sammlung von Robj ist daher eine Tapisserie französischen künstlerischen Talents der Art Deco Ära. Robj hat tatsächlich künstlerische Wettbewerbe unter den französischen Künstlern dieser Epoche geldlich unterstützt. Unter Robj's Designern findet man folgende Namen: Edouard Martin, Raoul Mabru, Pierre Toulgonat, Jean Courtebassis, Henri Martin, Jeanne Lavergne, Marthe Coulon und Georges Laurent. Was Robj-Objekte von vielen anderen Arten der dekorativen Kunst unterscheidet ist, dass sie die seltenste aller Attribute der Kunst verkörpern: Ein Gefühl für Humor und Charme. Robj-Objekte sind niemals schwerfällig, bedrückend ernsthaft oder grimmig - und deshalb wird ihre hohe künstlerische Qualität von einigen oft übersehen. Mit ihrer klaren Belegung des Art Deco Stils und in ihrer freimütigen Fähigkeit einer weltlichen Haushaltsfunktion zu dienen können Robj-Objekte den Beschauer verführen, meistens jedoch schon allein aufgrund ihrer charmanten Wunderlichkeit.

In *Art et Décoration* wurde die Pariser Gallerie, in welcher Robj gehandelt wurde, im Februar 1929 beschrieben. Sie wurde von dem Architekten und Designer René Herbst entworfen. Gemäss dem Bericht über Herbst's Entwurf war ihre Bestimmung einzigartig. "Robj's dekorative Objekte zeichnen sich durch zwei typische Merkmale aus: Ornamentale und funktionelle Keramik-Objekte auf der einen Seite und Beleuchtungsanlagen und -zubehör (Lampen, Nachtlichter, Parfüm-Lampen) auf der anderen. Deshalb war es wichtig, zwei verschiedene Bestandteile für die Gallerie zu übernehmen; Licht auf den ersten Teil zu werfen und die lichtgebende Kapazität des zweiten Typs zu unterstreichen, ohne gleichzeitig die Einheit des Ensembles zu brechen." Das Unternehmen benutzte das folgende Motto, welches heutzutage nicht weniger bedeutungsvoll ist: "Les bibelots Robj sont le complément de tout intérieur élégant" - oder: "Die Nippsachen von Robj vervollständigen jede elegante Inneneinrichtung."

Robj hat dekorative Figurinen produziert, deren einzige Funktion es war schön zu sein, aber gewöhnlicherweise befriedigen Robj-Objekte zusätzlich eine gebräuchliche Funktion. Oft besteht eine wunderliche und transparente Verbindung zwischen der Funktion des Objekts und seinem Entwurf. Zum Beispiel gibt es eine Parfüm-Lampe in Form eines Mönchs, der ein Weihrauchgefäss hält und verschiedene andere, welche Frauen darstellen, die Blumensträusse halten. Das Objekt teilt dem Betrachter seine Funktion mit. Unter den Robj-Objekten findet man eine Fülle der folgenden: Likörflaschen, Tintenfässer, Puderdosen, Bonbonniéren, Aschenbecher, Seifenschüsselchen, Videpoches, Buchstützen, Parfüm-Lampen, Cocktail-Shaker, Cremedosen, Marmeladengläser,

Lampen, Kuchen- und Käseglocken, Tee- und Kaffeekannen, Plätzchen- und Tabakdosen, Tassen und Untertassen, Zuckerdosen, Milchkännchen, Likörglashalter, Uhren, Thermometerhalter, Reibahlen, Wandmasken und viele andere Dinge. Die Likörflaschen waren in den Vereinigten Staaten sehr populär, möglicherweise aufgrund ihrer (ironischen) Verheimlichung des Alkohols; ein wichtiges Element in der Zeit der Prohibition. Robj produzierte auch Kunstglas in brillanten Farben sowie eine Reihe von kommerziellen Parfums (*Le Sécret du Robj* und *Entre Tous*), und eine grosse Variation aus Bronze und Kunstglas hergestellter Beleuchtungsgegenstände.

Robj fertigte eine beträchtliche Variation in Puderdosen aller Grössen an, einige sogar gross genug um eine kleine Flasche Whiskey darin zu verbergen. Typisch sind diese in der Form einer Frau mit einem sehr voluminösen Rock. Hierbei wurden viele verschiedene Designs benutzt. Porzellan eignete sich ideal für die Herstellung von Parfüm-Lampen, da es hoch lichtdurchlässig ist, wenn es von innen beleuchtet wird. Die Hitze des Lichts verhalf dem Parfüm sich schnell in die umgebende Luft zu verbreiten. Einige Parfüm-Lampen waren auch aus sehr feinem Kunstglas auf einem Bronze- oder Holzständer geformt. In diesen Fällen ist das Glas von sehr feiner Qualität und wurde oben mit einer Einbuchtung für das Parfüm versehen. Zum Ende des 20. Jahrhunderts hörte der Brauch von Parfüm-Lampen auf. Jedoch, die Idee des Parfümerhitzens, um es sich in der Luft verbreiten zu lassen, datiert zurück bis zum tatsächlichen Ursprung des Parfüms selbst, dessen Name wörtlich "durch den Rauch" heisst. Keines der Robj-Parfüme scheint einen grossen kommerziellen Erfolg gehabt zu haben, und alle sollten wahrscheinlich als relativ selten angesehen werden. In einigen Fällen, ca. 1928, wurden Robj-Parfüme (deren exakter Name interessant wäre zu wissen) in von Baccarat gefertigten Kristallflaschen abgefüllt, deren Stöpsel die Form einer Krone haben.

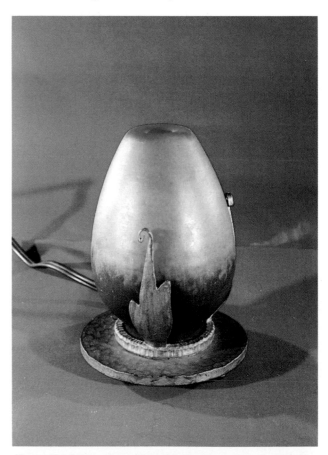

Figure 18. Robj perfume lamp of bronze and glass, a diminutive size model which glows brilliantly in blue and orange when lit.

Czechoslovakian Perfume Bottles: The Stunning Opaques

Flacons de Parfum Tchéchoslovaques: les Opaques Etonnants

Donna G. Sims

The country of Czechoslovakia was formed from the Czech and Slovak regions of Austria-Hungary, and included parts of what had been Bohemia. The Allied victors of World War I rewarded Czech and Slovak assistance during the war with the creation of Czechoslovakia as a sovereign country in 1918. After Germany absorbed the Sudetenland (German speaking) portion of Czechoslovakia in October 1938 and invaded greater Czechoslovakia in March 1939, the glass factories, about 600 in number, were converted to munitions production. Artists fled and glass-making skills that had been passed from generation to generation vanished, seemingly overnight. This confluence of events, the creation of Czechoslovakia in 1918 and the closure of the glass factories in the early years of the war, meant that even though the Bohemian region had been a glass-making center for centuries, the artistic glassware leaving it had the Czechoslovakian mark on it for only two decades. The beautiful Czechoslovakian perfume bottles made in that twenty-year period are appreciated and sought after by more and more collectors with each passing year.

When collectors think of Czechoslovakian perfume bottles, the image that most often comes to mind is that of a beautiful translucent bottle, clear or delicately colored, highly cut, and reflecting light in such a way as to give a shimmering appearance. But there is another category of Czech bottles of which some collectors are less aware: Opaque.

Opaque bottles are ones which are impervious to light; light cannot pass through. Heinrich Hoffman and Henry Schlevogt (under the name of Ingrid in honor of his young daughter), designed and produced some of the world's most beautiful perfume bottles.

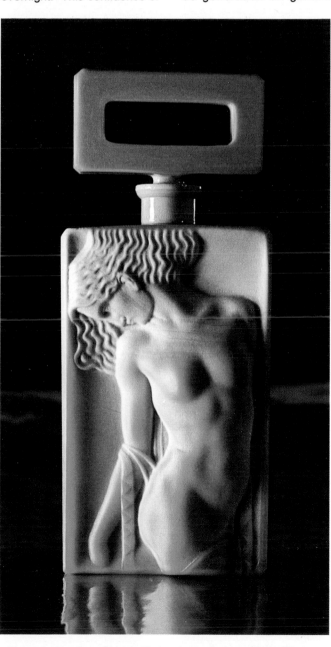

Figure 1. Czech perfume bottle in opaque aqua, molded with a sea nymph on the front. Collection of Donna Sims.

La Tchéchoslovaquie (aujourd'hui la République Tchèque et la Slovaquie) a été formée à partir des territoires tchèques et slovaques et comprenait des régions ayant fait partie de l'Autriche et de la Hongrie. Les Alliés, vainqueurs de la Première Guerre Mondiale récompensèrent l'aide des Tchèques et des Slovaques pendant la guerre en créant l'état souverain tchéchoslovaque en 1918. Après que le Troisième Reich ait absorbé la Sudetenland en octobre 1938 et envahie la Tchéchoslovaquie même en mars 1939, les usines de verre, au nombre de 600, se mirent à produire des munitions. Les artistes s'enfuirent et des techniques transmises de génération en génération disparurent du jour au lendemain. La suite de ces événements, la création de l'état tchéchoslovaque en 1918 et la fermeture des usines de verre au début de la guerre firent qu'en dépit d'une tradition multiséculaire de l'industrie du verre de la Bohème, le verre ne porta la marque de la Tchéchoslovaquie que pendant vingt ans. Les magnifiques flacons de parfum tchèques produits pendant cette brève période sont appréciés et recherchés par un nombre croissant de collectionneurs.

Lorsque les collectionneurs pensent aux flacons de parfum tchèques, l'image première est celle d'un beau flacon translucide, clair ou d'une couleur délicate, très travaillée, et avec des reflets qui lui donnent une apparence irridescente. Mais il existe une autre catégorie de flacons tchèques que certains collectionneurs ont moins à l'esprit: opaque.

Les flacons opaques sont faits de verre imperméables à la lumière; la lumière ne peut pas passer. Heinrich Hoffman et Henry Schlevogt (sous le nom "Ingrid" en hommage à sa fille) dessinèrent et produisirent des flacons de parfum qui sont parmi les plus beaux du monde. Ils découvrirent des procédés

They developed methods of producing glass which give the appearance of semi-precious stones and other natural creations complete with gradations of color. The marbling of these glass products is nearly indistinguishable from their natural counterparts. Nearly all opaque colors are Hoffman or Schlevogt designs and are marked with either the Hoffman butterfly or the Ingrid signature.

There are fourteen known colors of Czechoslovakian opaque perfume bottles and accessories that emulate nature's creations. All are scarce, but many are quite rare. Experts agree that the most frequently seen opaque color is black, also referred to as jet or onyx. Opaque green (malachite) and opaque blue (lapis lazuli) rank second and third. The rest of the colors are seen less often and some are exceedingly rare. In no particular order, they are opaque aqua (turquoise), opaque light brown (light brown agate), opaque dark brown (dark brown agate), opaque pink (light pink coral), ivory (ivory), opaque green (bright green jade), opaque red (red coral), opaque orange (orange coral), opalescent (opal), jade (the most common shade of green jade), and opaque deep red (garnet). A handful of bottles combined two or even three opaque colors.

Examples shown are some of the most desirable Czechoslovakian perfume bottles sought by collectors. The first example is opaque aqua, representing the natural stone turquoise. At 7-3/4" high, its size alone distinguishes it. The sea nymph on the front is one of the most sensuous and detailed nudes seen on perfume bottles. The combination of size, color, and detailing of the nude put this Ingrid-signed perfume in a category all its own.

Black, the most common opaque color, is an imitation of jet or onyx and is usually seen with a different color stopper, most commonly clear or frosted clear. Stoppers in pink, pink coral, amethyst, red, red coral, green, malachite, ivory, and amber have also been seen with black bottles. The example shown combines the simple, but elegant, black bottle with a three-dimensional nude stopper. The nude is partially draped and rests atop the bottle with one leg tucked under her and the other draped over the bottle. The understated elegance of this bottle is unequaled. It is 6-1/2" high and is acid-etched Made in Czechoslovakia.

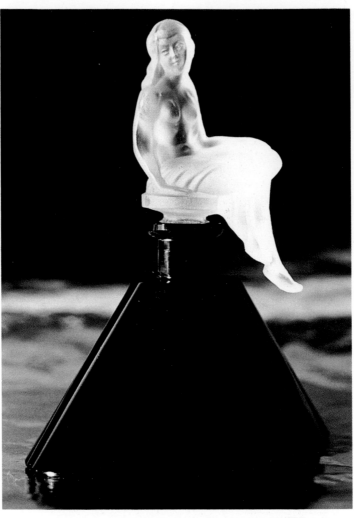

Figure 2. Czech perfume bottle in opaque black; stopper is in frosted crystal. Collection of Donna Sims.

de fabrication donnant au verre un aspect de pierres semi-précieuses et d'autres créations naturelles avec une gamme complète de coloris. Les marbrures de ces verres sont très difficiles à distinguer de leurs modèles naturels. Presque toutes les couleurs opaques sont des conceptions de Hoffman ou Schlevogt et sont frappées du papillon de Hoffman ou de la signature 'Ingrid'.

Il y a quatorze couleurs opaques de flacons de parfums et d'accessoires de verre tchécoslovaques. Tous sont difficiles à trouver, et certaines sont rares. Les experts s'accordent sur le fait que la couleur opaque la plus répandue est le noir, appelée aussi onyx. Le vert opaque (malachite) et le bleu opaque (lapis lazuli) sont en seconde et troisième positions. Les autres couleurs se rencontrent moins souvent et certaines sont très rares. Enumérées sans ordre elles sont: aqua opaque (turquoise), marron clair opaque (agate marron clair), marron foncé opaque (agate marron foncé), rose opaque (corail rose clair), ivoire (ivoire), vert opaque (jade vert vif), rouge opaque (corail rouge), orange opaque (corail orange), opalescent (opale), jade (le ton le plus fréquent de jade), et rouge foncé opaque (grenat). Seule une poignée de flacons sont composés de deux ou trois couleurs opaques.

Les exemples cités ici sont parmi les plus recherchés par les collectionneurs de flacons de parfums tchèques. Le premier est aqua opaque, imitant la turquoise naturelle. Sa taille d'environ 20cm suffit à la rendre exceptionelle. La nymphe aquatique sur la face est un des nus les plus sensuels et les plus détaillés figurant sur un flacon de parfum. La combinaison de taille, couleur et dessin du nu vaut à ce flacon de parfum Ingrid un classement à part.

Le noir, la couleur opaque la plus fréquente, est une imitation de l'onyx et se trouve le plus souvent assorti d'un bouchon d'une autre couleur, de préférence sans couleur ou sans couleur dépolie. Mais il existe aussi des bouchons roses, rose corail, améthystes, rouges, rouge corail, malachites, ivoires, et ambres avec des flacons noirs. Cet example allie le flacon noir simple mais élégant avec un nu sculpté pour bouchon. Le nu est partiellement couvert et juché sur le flacon, assis sur une de ses jambes et l'autre

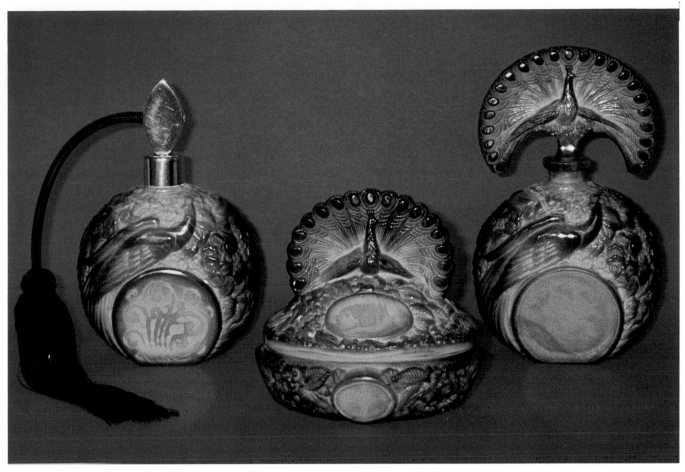

Figure 3. Czech perfume bottle set in malachite [opaque green] with a peacock motif. Collection of Lanette Martin.

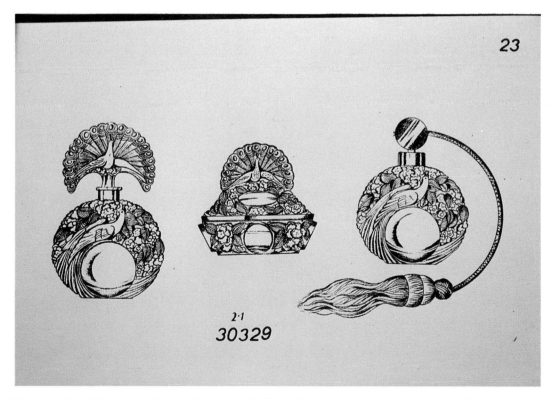

Figure 4. The original page, showing the set seen in Figure 3, from a salesman's sample folder of Ingrid designs.
Collection of Donna Sims.

After black, green is the opaque color most often seen. It is an imitation of nature's malachite stone. Several styles of malachite bottles were made in dresser sets, but finding one completely intact is no easy task. The example shown is such a set, as is evidenced by a copy of item number 30329, page number 23, from a representative's sample folder of Ingrid designs. This very unusual design has a peacock in its full glory as the stopper for the perfume bottle and as the handle for the powder box. The powder box is 5 inches, the atomizer is 7" and the perfume bottle is 7-5/8" high. This is an example of superb creativity and execution of design.

Even though opaque blue, an imitation of lapis lazuli, is the third most common opaque color, it is still difficult to find. The example shown has a nude on the front of the bottle and two nudes on the stopper. The nudes on the stopper were designed so that a leg of each nude forms the tiara stopper. The exceptional marbling and gradation of color on this lapis lazuli bottle greatly enhance this magnificent design. It is 6" high and is signed Ingrid.

Opaque light brown and opaque dark brown are imitations of light brown agate and dark brown agate. These two colors have only been seen together. The powder box shown has an opaque light brown base with an opaque dark brown top. Even the nude handle on the powder box has gradations of color. It is 4-1/4" high and is a Hoffman design.

Opaque red, an imitation of red coral, is one of the most beautiful opaque colors. The bottle shown has a leaping gazelle on its front and is molded all over its surface with flowers, continuing even on the bottom of the bottle forming four small feet. The large molded flower stopper has gradations of red shading to yellow. This rare red perfume bottle is 6-1/2" high and is acid-etched Made in Czechoslovakia.

Opaque pale pink, an imitation of angel-skin coral, is a color so scarce that it has been seen only as

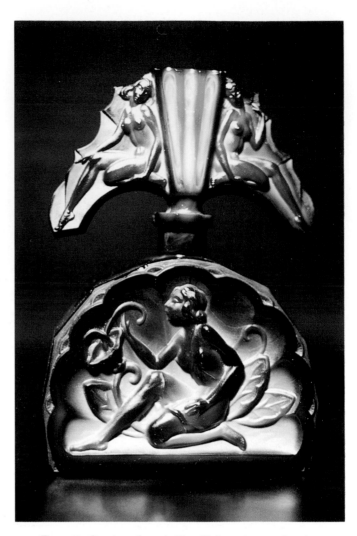

Figure 5. Czech perfume bottle with tiara stopper of nudes in opaque blue, lapis lazuli. Collection of Stephen Kraynak.

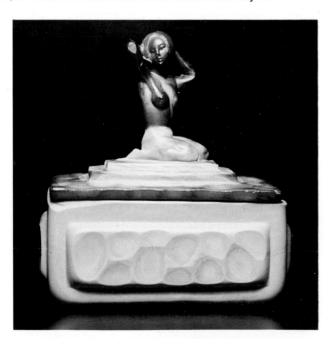

Figure 6. Czech crystal powder box in opaque light and dark brown. Colleciton of Donna Sims.

disposée au-dessus du flacon. L'élégance discrète de ce flacon est inégalée.

Après le noir, le vert est la couleur opaque la plus répandue. C'est une imitation de la malachite naturelle. Plusieurs styles de flacons de malachite furent produits avec des nécessaires de toilette, mais il est bien difficile d'en trouver qui soit complet. L'exemple ici en est un, comme le montre une copie de l'article 30329, page 23, d'un dépliant de vendeur de la marque Ingrid. Cette conception inhabituelle est dominée par un paon dans toute sa gloire comme bouchon du flacon de parfum et comme poignée du poudrier. C'est un exemple de créativité et d'exécution superbes.

Même si le bleu opaque, une imitation du lapis lazuli, est au troisième rang de production de couleurs opaques, il est encore difficile à trouver. L'exemple ici a un nu sur la face du flacon et deux nus sur le bouchon. Les nus du bouchon sont conçus de manière à ce qu'une jambe de chaque nu produise un bouchon en tiare. La marbrure et la gradation de couleur de ce flacon lapis lazuli rehaussent considérablement son dessin magnifique. Le marron

a stopper. The example shown has the Hoffman shell-like design on the black bottle, with a pale pink coral stopper. It is 4-1/8" high and is marked with the Hoffman cameo butterfly.

Ivory is very rare in opaque perfumes. It replicates one of nature's most precious and most desired natural creations. Perfume bottles with nudes in relief are sought after with a special determination by collectors. This exquisite ivory bottle with beautiful detailed nudes dancing all around the base is a treasure. The red and ivory combination is, at the same time, both sophisticated and breathtaking. The ivory color, its combination with red, and the detailed nudes all combine to make this an extremely rare and desirable bottle. Ivory has been seen in combinations with black, red, red coral, and lapis. This bottle is 8" high and is marked Ingrid.

The black atomizer with the red nudes is a two-color bottle. It is the same design as the ivory bottle and is indicative of Henry Schlevogt's design genius. The same beautiful design takes on a completely different appearance when produced in other colors. This bottle is stunning with the vivid contrast of the red nudes against the black background. It is 7-1/4" high and is marked Ingrid.

Another opaque green differs from malachite; it imitates a scarce color of jade, bright green, sometimes referred to as green-apple jade. This Hoffman columnar design was made in many colors, in three known sizes, and with at least five different stoppers. At four inches high, this example is

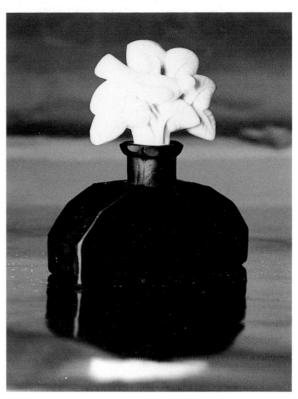

Figure 8. Czech perfume bottle in opaque black with a stopper in opaque pink, by Hoffman. Collection of Donna Sims.

opaque clair et foncé sont des imitations de l'agate marron clair et foncé. Même la poignée en forme de nu du poudrier a des gradations de couleur. Le rouge opaque, une imitation du corail rouge, est une des plus belles couleurs opaques. Le flacon en exposition a une gazelle bondissante sur sa face et des fleurs moulées sur toute sa surface qui débordent sur le bas formant quatre petits pieds. Le bouchon en forme de grande fleur a des nuances de rouge allant jusqu'au jaune. Le rose pâle opaque, une imitation de corail, est une couleur si rare qu'elle n'est connue que sous forme de bouchon. L'exemple ici est un dessin style Hoffman en forme de coquille sur le flacon noir avec un bouchon de corail rose pâle.

Des flacons de parfum en ivoire, une des matières naturelles les plus recherchées, sont très rares. Ce flacon exquis avec des nus aux détails élégants dansant tout autour de la base est un trésor. La couleur ivoire, en combinaison avec le rouge, et les nus élégants conspirent à en faire un flacon très rare et désirable. L'ivoire a été produit assorti de noir, de rouge, de rouge corail, et de lapis.

L'atomiseur noir avec les nus est un flacon bicolore. Il présente le même dessin que le flacon en ivoire et montre le génie créatif de Henry Schlevogt. Le même beau dessin donne un effet complètement différent exécuté dans d'autres couleurs. Le contraste des nus rouges sur le fond noir de ce flacon est frappant.

Il existe un autre vert opaque différent de la malachite; il imite une couleur rare de jade, le vert

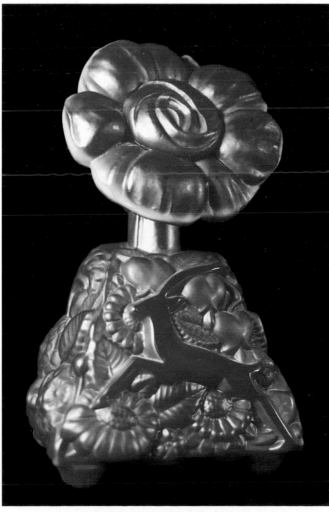

Figure 7. Czech perfume bottle in opaque red. Collection of Stephen Kraynak.

the smallest size. It is marked with the Hoffman cameo butterfly.

Opaque coral is a nearly perfect visual replication of natural orange coral. The example shown is a Heinrich Hoffman bottle and is marked with the Hoffman cameo butterfly. It also incorporates a style seen in four examples of colors in this article, that of a shell effect. Every known example with this shell effect design is a Hoffman bottle. There are two nudes on the front of the coral bottle and two on the back. The stopper has delicate birds in flight and has shade gradations from coral to yellow. The elements of rare color and nudes combine to make this bottle very desirable. It is 4-3/4" high.

Hoffman used his designs with different stoppers and produced them in different colors. The tricolor bottle pictured is the same design as the orange coral example. It is evident that when Hoffman varied the colors, he didn't simply make a blue, a red, and a coral one. Each bottle was a creation and these two bottles, while the same design, look quite different because of the different colors, finishes on the bottles, and different stoppers. The tricolor combination and especially the design of the stopper give the bottle an Egyptian look. The opening of Tutankhamen's tomb in the 1920's was the inspiration for many works of art including, most

vif, connu aussi sous le nom de vert pomme. Ce dessin de Hoffman en forme de colonne a été produit en plusieurs couleurs, en trois tailles connues, avec au moins cinq bouchons différents. Haut de 10 cm cet exemple est le plus petit. Le plus grand est frappé du papillon en camée de Hofmman, contrairement au moyen et petit.

L'opaque corail est une reproduction presque parfaite du corail orange naturel. L'exemple illustré est un flacon de Heinrich Hoffman portant la marque du papillon Hoffman en camée. Il comprend également un style que l'on retrouve dans trois exemples de couleurs dans cet article, en coquille. Tout exemple connu de ce style coquillage est un flacon Hoffman. Il y a deux nus sur le front du flacon en corail et deux sur le dos. Le bouchon a des oiseaux délicats en vol et des nuances de couleur allant du corail au jaune.

Hoffman assortissait ses conceptions de différents bouchons et les produisait dans des couleurs différentes. Il est évident que quand Hoffman variait les couleurs il ne créait pas simplement une en bleue, une en rouge en et une en corail. Chaque flacon est une création particulière et ces deux flacons, quoique de la même conception, semblent très différents grâce à leurs couleurs différentes, à la finition des flacons, et aux bouchons différents. La combinaison tricolore, et surtout le dessin du bouchon, donnent au flacon un air égyptien.

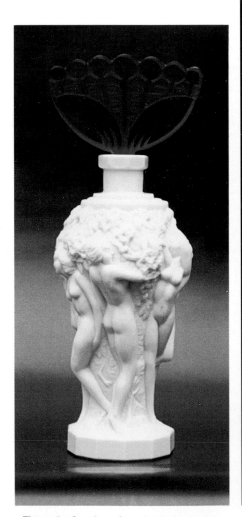

Figure 9. Czech perfume bottle in opaque ivory with a red crystal stopper. Collection of Marianne Franke.

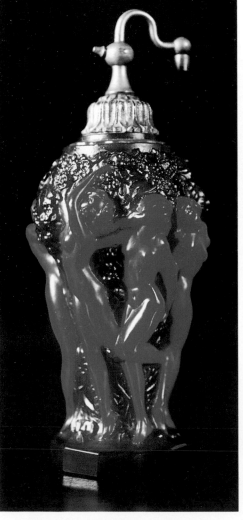

Figure 10. Czech perfume atomizer in red and black opaque crystal. Collection of Ruth Forsythe.

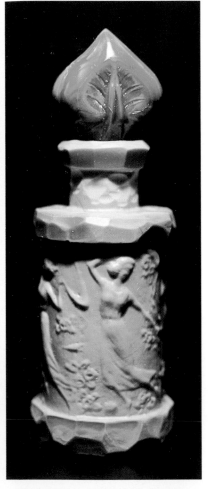

Figure 11. Czech perfume bottle in opaque bright green jade. Collection of Ruth Forsythe.

likely, this design. This tricolor bottle is 4-1/4" high and is marked with the Hoffman cameo butterfly.

The recent discovery of two bottles with an Oriental appearance has added another dimension to the Czechoslovakian bottles. One has a combination of the colors of garnet and red coral. The other has the combination of the colors of the most common shade of green jade combined with orange coral accents, with a flat polished garnet atop its stopper. Garnet, red coral, green jade and orange coral have been used in the making of Chinese jewelry and other types of Chinese art for centuries. Both are 3" high. The garnet bottle is acid-etched Made in Czechoslovakia.

Opalescent is an imitation of the semi-precious opal gem. Light plays off of this color as light does off of an opal; it is even fiery like an opal. The opalescent powder box shown has as its handle three Muses playing musical instruments. It is 4-3/4" high and is signed Ingrid.

In recent years, the Czechoslovakian perfume bottles and accessories have begun to be recognized and appreciated for the art objects that they truly are. They were thoughtfully designed and those designs were carefully executed, as is evidenced by the bottles in this article and in particular by the bottles that are the same styles but different colors. The bottle pictured in three colors - red coral, lapis, and malachite - represents Leda of the mythological characters Leda and the Swan. It demonstrates several facts. First, the bottles were individually hand-finished, not mass produced on an assembly line. The three Ledas are all slightly different heights, and this variance is not only in the total height of the bottles, but they differ at every point on the bottle from the base up to the lip; they vary in size from 6-1/4" to 6-1/2" high. The stoppers cannot be switched as they were all apparently hand-seated by the emeri-ground method. Second, opaque colors were not always paired with a matching opaque stopper; some were made with specially designed clear ones. These three bottles are perfect examples to validate this. The design of the flowers on the stoppers of the red and green bottles duplicate perfectly the flower design down the sides of the bottle. It is obvious the combination is correct. Third, these bottles were carefully designed. Pictured is an original blueprint of this bottle, discovered only recently and rescued as it was about to be forever lost in a fire. Since the bottle shows only

La découverte du tombeau de Toutankhamon dans les années 20 a été l'inspiration de nombreuses oeuvres d'art et dans celle-ci selon toute vraisemblance. Ce flacon tricolore de 11 cm de hauteur est frappé de la marque du papillon en camée de Hoffman.

La découverte récente de deux flacons d'apparence orientale a ajouté une autre dimension aux flacons tchèques. Un comprend une combinaison des couleurs grenat et corail rouge. L'autre est composé du vert jade le plus courant avec des accents de corail orange, avec un grenat plat poli sur le bouchon. Le grenat, corail rouge, jade vert et corail orange sont utilisés en bijouterie et dans les autres arts chinois depuis des siècles. L'opaline est une imitation de l'opale, pierre semi-précieuse. La lumière a les mêmes effets sur cette couleur que la lumière sur l'opale; elle est même fulgurante comme l'opale. La poignée du poudrier opaline illustré comprend trois muses jouant des instruments musicaux.

Récemment, les flacons de parfum et accessoires tchèques ont retenu l'attention qu'ils méritent en tant qu'oeuvres d'art qu'ils ont toujours été. Leur conception était aussi soigné que leur exécution, ainsi que le prouvent les flacons de cet article, et en particulier les flacons de même conception mais de couleurs différentes. Le flacon illustré en trois couleurs, corail rouge, lapis et malachite, représente Leda du couple mythologique de Leda et du cygne. Il démontre plusieurs faits. Premièrement, que les flacons furent terminés à la main et non pas sur une chaîne de fabrication. Les trois Ledas sont de tailles différentes et cette variation n'est pas seulement dans la hauteur mais dans toutes les dimensions du haut en bas; elles varient de 15,8 cm à 16,5 cm. Les bouchons ne peuvent être interchangés étant donné qu'ils ont été ajustés à la main à l'émeri. Deuxièmement, les couleurs opaques ne sont pas toujours assorties d'un bouchon opaque correspondant; plusieurs ont des bouchons translucides spécialement conçus. Ces trois flacons en sont un exemple parfait. Le dessin des fleurs sur les bouchons rouge et vert reproduisent parfaitement le dessin des fleurs le long des côtés du flacon. Il est évident que cette combinaison est correcte. Troisièmement, les flacons ont été soigneusement conçus. Le dessin de fabrication de ce flacon, découvert tout récemment alors qu'il allait être consigné aux flammes

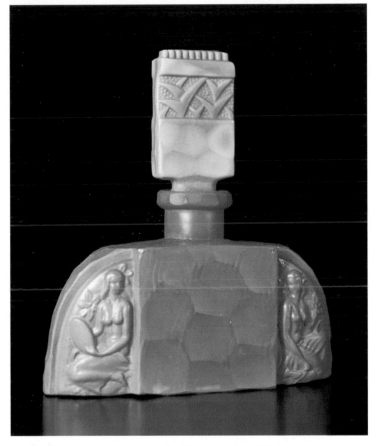

Figure 12. Czech perfume bottle in opaque coral, by Hoffman. Collection of Donna Sims.

a beautiful nude, it would be speculation to call her Leda. However, the matching powder box clearly shows that she is Leda because of the appearance of the Swan on the powder box lid. Fourth, the original blueprint pictured shows that stoppers and bottles were individually designed, and then combined and given a combination design number. For the Leda bottle shown in three colors, the bottle was design number 513, and the stopper number 621, with the combination of these two as design number 52678. The matching powder box shows that the base is design number 565 and the lid is number 566, with the combination of the pair as design number 1079. Fifth, as is also evident from the blueprint, the stopper shown is not the same design as the stoppers of the three examples. The creators of the Czech perfume bottles, in many cases, designed more than one stopper for each base and vice versa.

While beautiful works of art in glass are certainly being designed and crafted in various parts of the world today, the unique artistry demonstrated by the Bohemians reached its zenith in the form of Czechoslovakian perfume bottles during the two decades between this century's two world wars. During this brief period of history, Czechoslovakian artists and craftsmen created treasures that are being appreciated by more and more collectors with each passing day.

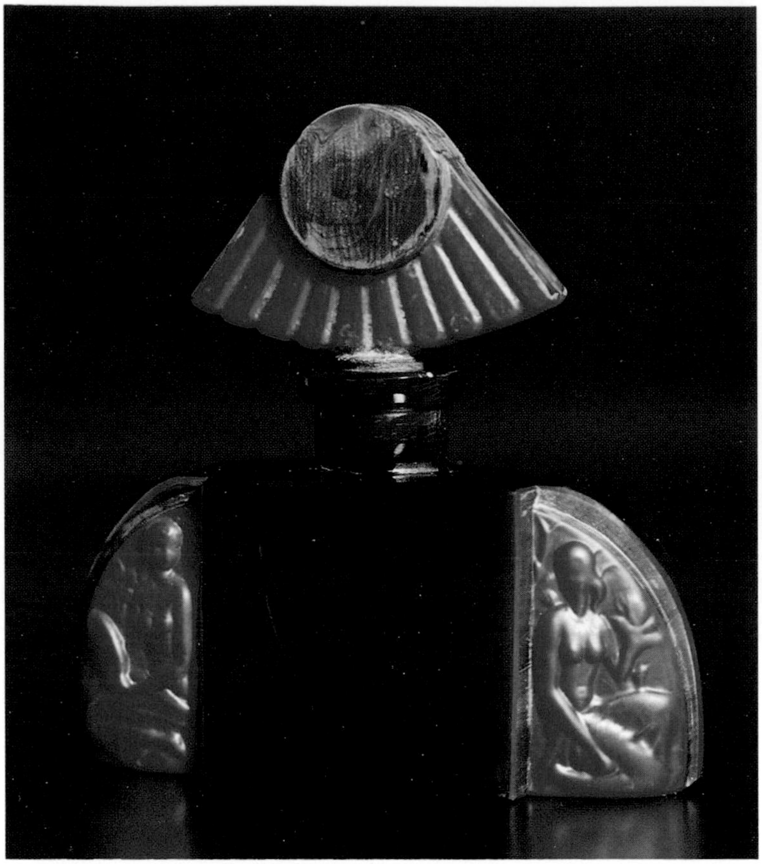

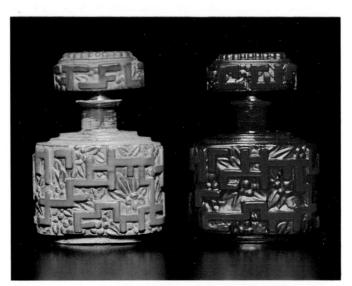

Figure 13. Czech perfume bottle in three colors: opaque red, green, black, by Hoffman. Collection of Ruth Forsythe.

Figure 14. Czech perfume bottles in opaque garnet and red coral, and in green jade and orange coral.
Collection of Ken Leach and Richard Peters, Gallery 47.

est illustré. Il ne serait pas possible de conclure du seul beau nu sur le devant du flacon qu'il s'agit de Leda. Mais le couvercle du poudrier assorti montre clairement qu'il s'agit de Leda grâce au cygne s'y trouvant. Quatrièmement, le dessin de fabrication d'origine montre que les flacons et les bouchons étaient conçus ensemble, puis assortis et un numéro de fabrication combiné attribué. Pour le flacon de Leda en trois couleurs, le flacon était le dessin numéro 513 et le bouchon était le dessin numéro 621 et la combinaison des deux était le dessin numéro 52678. Le poudrier assorti montre que la base est celle du dessin numéro 565 et le couvercle celui du dessin numéro 566, alors que les deux ensembles sont le dessin 1079. Cinquièmement, et toujours du dessin, le bouchon n'est pas du même dessin que les bouchons des trois exemples. Dans de nombreux cas, les créateurs de flacons de parfums tchèques déssinaient plus d'un bouchon pour chaque flacon et *vice versa*.

Alors que de nos jours on crée des oeuvres d'art en verre dans diverses parties du globe, l'art unique que nous offrent les artistes de la Bohème atteignit son zénith dans les flacons de parfum tchèques pendant les vingt années de l'entre deux guerres. Cette périod vit la création de trésors recherchés par un nombre croissant de collectionneurs.

Correspondence for the author may be addressed to: Donna G. Sims, PO Box 187, Galena, Ohio 43021.

Tschechoslowakische Parfümflaschen
Die überwaltigenden Opaques (Undurchsichtigen)

Die Tschechoslowakei wurde aus den tschechischen und slowakischen Regionen Böhmens gegründet und beinhaltete auch österreichische Teile. Die alliierten Sieger des 1. Weltkriegs gewährten den Tschechen und Slowaken Hilfe während des Krieges mit der Gründung der Tschechoslowakei als souveränem Staat in 1918. Nachdem Deutschland das deutschprechende Sudetenland, Teil der Tschechoslowakei, im Oktober 1938 eingenommen und die Gross-Tschechoslowakei angegriffen hatte, wurden die Glasfabriken, ca. 600 an der Zahl, in Munitionsproduktionen umgewandelt. Künstler flüchteten und das Geschick der Glasherstellung, welches von Generation zu Generation überliefert wurde, verschwand scheinbar über Nacht. Das Zusammentreffen der Ereignisse, die Gründung der Tschechoslowakei in 1918 und die Schliessung der Glasfabriken in den frühen Jahren des Krieges, bedeutete, dass das tschechoslowakische Kennzeichen sein Merkmal auf den das Land verlassenden Glasprodukten nur für zwei Dekaden hinterliess, obwohl die böhmische Region seit Jahrzehnten ein Glasherstellungszentrum war. Die wunderschönen tschechoslowakischen Parfümflaschen, die in dieser kurzen zwanzigjährigen Periode entstanden, werden von mehr und mehr Sammlern mit jedom vorübergohondon Jahr mehr bewundert und begehrt.

Wenn Sammler an tschechoslowakische Parfümflaschen denken, ist die Vorstellung davon in den meisten Fällen die einer schönen lichtdurchlässigen Flasche, klar oder zart gefärbt, erhaben geschliffen und das Licht in einer Art reflektierend, die eine schimmernde Erscheinung erzeugt. Aber es gibt auch eine andere Kategorie tschechischer Flaschen, die einigen Sammlern nicht so bekannt ist: Opaque. Opake Flaschen sind aus für Licht undurchdringlichem Glas, Licht kann nicht hindurchscheinen. Heinrich Hoffman und Henry Schlevogt (unter dem Namen "Ingrid" zur Ehre seiner jungen Tochter) entwarfen und produzierten einige der Welt schönsten Parfümflaschen. Sie entwickelten Methoden Glas herzustellen, das das Aussehen von Halbedelsteinen und anderen natürlichen Schöpfungen in kompletter Farbabstufung hatte. Die Marmorierung dieser Glasprodukte ist fast nicht von deren natürlichen Gegenstücken zu unterscheiden. Fast alle opake Farben sind Hoffman und Schlevogt Designs und entweder mit dem Hoffmann Schmetterling oder der Ingrid-Signatur gekennzeichnet.

Es gibt vierzehn bekannte Farben tschechoslowakischer opaker Parfümflaschen und Accessoires. Sie sind alle spärlich, aber die meisten sehr selten. Experten sind sich einig, dass die am häufigsten vorkommende opake Farbe schwarz ist, auch auf "Jet" oder Onyx verweisbar. Opak-grün (Malachit) und opak-blau (Lapislazuli) rangieren an zweiter und dritter Stelle. Die restlichen Farben sieht man weniger und einige sind äusserst selten. Sie

sind, in keiner speziellen Reihenfolge: Opak-aquamarin (Türkis), opak-hellbraun (hellbrauner Achat), opak-dunkelbraun (dunklebrauner Achat), opak-rosa (hellrosa Koralle), elfenbein (Elfenbein), opak-grün (leuchtend grüner Jade), opak-rot (rote Koralle), opak-orange (orangene Koralle), opalisierend (Opal), jade-blassgrün (die bekannteste Schattierung grüner Jade) und opak-dunkelrot (Granat). Eine Handvoll von Flaschen kombinierte zwei oder sogar drei opaker Farben.

Beispiele, die hier gezeigt werden, sind einige der von Sammlern am meistbegehrten tschechoslowakischer Parfümflaschen. Das erste Beispiel ist opak-aquamarin, den Naturstein Türkis verkörpernd. Mit einer Höhe von 7 3/4 inches kennzeichnet dies allein schon seine Grösse. Die Wassernymphe auf der Vorderseite ist eine der sinnlichsten und detailgetreuesten Aktfiguren, die man auf einer Parfümflasche je gesehen hat. Die Kombination aus Grösse, Farbe und detaillierter Nacktheit stellte dieses, Ingrid-signierte Parfüm, in eine für sich eigene Kategorie.

Schwarz, die gebräuchlichste opake Farbe, ist eine Imitation von Jet oder Onyx und wird gewöhnlicherweise mit einem andersfarbigen Stöpsel gefunden, der meistens durchsichtig oder mattglasig ist. Auch sah man Stöpsel in den Farben rosa, rosa-korall, amethyst, rot, rot-korall, grün, malachit, elfenbein und bernstein mit schwarzen Flaschen. Das gezeigte Beispiel kombiniert die einfache aber elegante schwarze Flasche mit einem dreidimensionalen Stöpsel einer nackten Figur. Der Akt ist teilweise bedeckt und ruht oben auf der Flasche mit einem untergeschlagenem Bein, während das andere über die Flasche drapiert ist. Die zurückhaltende Eleganz dieser Flasche ist unvergleichlich.

Nach schwarz ist grün die am häufigsten vorkommende opake Farbe.

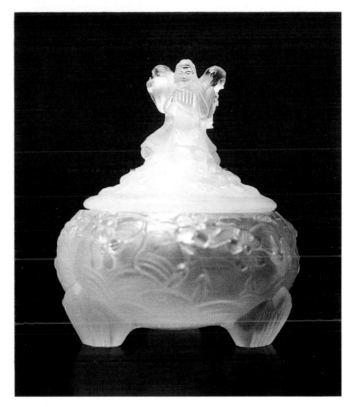

Figure 15. Czech powder jar in opalescent crystal.
Collection of Donna Sims.

Sie ist eine Imitation des Natursteins Malachit. Mehrer Arten solcher Malachit-Flaschen wurden als Toilettentisch-Garnituren gefertigt, aber nur eine davon komplett oder unversehrt zu finden ist keine leichte Sache. Das gezeigte Beispiel ist solch eine Garnitur, wie durch Posten Nr. 30329, Seiten-Nr. 23 einer Kopie einer Mustermappe eines Handelsvertreters von Ingrid-Designs bewiesen ist. Dieser sehr aussergewöhnliche Entwurf hat einen Pfau in seiner vollen Pracht als Stöpsel der Parfümflasche und als Griff der Puderdose. Es ist ein Beispiel von hervorragender Schaffenskraft und Entwurfsausführung.

Obwohl opak-blau, eine Imitation von Lapislazuli, die drittgebräuchliste opake Farbe ist, ist sie trotzalledem schwer zu finden. Das gezeigte Beispiel hat eine Aktfigur auf der Vorderseite der Flasche und zwei nackte Figuren auf dem Stöpsel. Die Aktfiguren auf dem Stöpsel wurden so gestaltet, dass ein Bein jeder Figur den Tiara-Stöpsel formt. Die ausserordentliche Marmorierung und Farbabstufung auf dieser Lapislazuli-Flasche steigern sehr

deutlich ihr prächtiges Design. Opak-hellbraun und opak-dunkelbraun sind Imitationen von hell- und dunkelbraunem Achat. Sogar der aktfigürliche Griff der Puderdose hat Abstufungen in Farbe. Opak-rot, eine Imitation von roter Koralle, ist eine der allerschönsten Opak-Farben. Die gezeigte Flasche hat eine springende Gazelle auf ihrer Vorderseite und ist auf ihrer gesamten Oberfläche mit Blumen geformt, bis hin zum Boden der Flasche, wo vier kleine Füsse gestaltet sind. Der grosse, modulierte Blumenstöpsel hat Farbabstufungen schattierend von rot bis hin zu gelb. Opak-blassrosa, eine Imitation von Engelshaut-Koralle, ist eine so seltene Farbe, dass man sie nur in einem Stöpsel finden konnte. Das gezeigte Beispiel hat auf der schwarzen Flasche das Hoffman muschelähnliche Design mit einem blassrosa Korallen-Stöpsel.

Elfenbein ist in Opak-Parfümen sehr selten. Es gibt eine der Natur kostbarsten und meistbegehrtesten Schöpfungen wieder. Diese exquisite Elfenbeinflasche mit wunderschön detaillierten Aktfiguren, die um den unteren Teil der Flasche herumtanzen, ist ein wahrer Schatz. Die Elfenbeinfarbe, ihre Kombination mit rot und die detaillierten Aktfiguren tragen alle dazu bei, sie zu einer extrem raren und begehrenswerten Flasche zu machen. Elfenbein

naturechter Orange-Koralle. Das Beispiel zeigt eine Heinrich Hoffman Flasche, die mit der Schmetterling-Kamee gekennzeichnet ist. Sie vereinigt auch einen Stil, der in drei Farbbeispielen dieses Artikels zu sehen ist, dem eines Muscheleffekts. Jedes bekannte Beispiel mit diesem Muscheleffekt-Entwurf ist eine Hoffman Flasche. Es befinden sich je zwei Aktfiguren auf der Vorder- und der Hinterseite der korallfarbenen Flasche. Der Stöpsel zeigt zierliche Vögel im Flug, mit Farbabstufungen von korall bis gelb.

Hoffmann gebrauchte seine Entwürfe mit verschiedenen Stöpseln und produzierte sie in verschiedenen Farben. Die abgebildete dreifarbige Flasche ist der gleiche Entwurf wie das orange-korallene Beispiel. Es ist offensichtlich, dass Hoffman nicht nur einfach eine blaue, eine rote oder eine korallfarbene machte, wenn er Farben variierte. Jede Flasche war eine eigene Kreation, und diese beiden Flaschen sehen wegen der verschiedenen Farben, den Ausarbeitungen auf der Flasche und der verschiedenen Stöpsel sehr verschieden voneinander aus, obwohl der gleiche Entwurf benutzt wurde. Die dreifarbige Kombination, und besonders der Entwurf des Stöpsels, geben der Flasche ein ägyptisches Aussehen. Tut-ench-Amun's Graböffnung in den 20er Jahren gab die Inspiration für viele Kunstarten, einschliesslich sehr

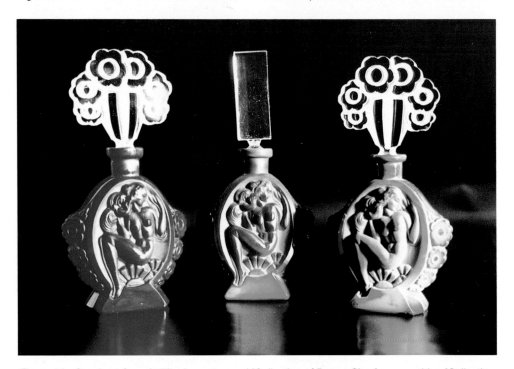

Figure 16. Czech perfume bottles in opaque red [Collection of Donna Sims]; opaque blue [Collection of Lisa Schwartz]; and opaque green [Collection of Lanette Martin].

wurde in der Kombination mit schwarz, rot, rot-korall und lapisfarben gefunden.

Der schwarze Zerstäuber mit den roten Aktfiguren ist eine zweifarbige Flasche. Es ist der gleiche Entwurf wie die Elfenbeinflasche und ist bezeichnend für Henry Schlevogt's Designer Genie. Derselbe schöne Entwurf nimmt eine völlig andere Erscheinung an, wenn er in anderen Farben produziert wird. Aufgrund ihres lebhaften Kontrasts zwischen den roten Aktfiguren und dem schwarzen Hintergrund ist diese Flasche betäubend schön.

Eine andere opak-grüne Farbe unterscheidet sich von malachit-farben; sie imitiert einen seltenen Farbton von Jade, hellgrün, manchmal auch als apfelgrüne Jade bezeichnet. Dieser säulenförmige Hoffman-Entwurf wurde in vielen Farben hergestellt, in drei bekannten Grössen und mit mindestens fünf verschiedenen Stöpseln. Mit einer Grösse von 4 inches ist dies das kleinste Beispiel. Die grösste Ausführung ist mit der Schmnetterling-Kamee von Hoffman markiert, die kleine und mittlere jedoch nicht.

Opak-korall ist fast eine perfekte visuelle Wiedergabe von

wahrscheinlich dieses Flaschenentwurfs. Die dreifarbige Flasche ist 4 1/4 inches hoch und mit der Schmetterling-Kamee von Hoffman markiert.

Die jüngste Entdeckung zweier Flaschen mit einem orientalischen Aussehen fügte den tschechoslowakischen Flaschen eine weitere Dimension bei. Eine davon hat eine Kombination der Farben granatrot und rot-korall. Die andere zeigt die Farbkombination der meist gebräuchlichsten Nuance von grüner Jade, verbunden mit orange-korallenen Abstufungen und hat einen flachen polierten Granat auf ihrem Stöpsel. Granatrot, rot-korall, jadegrün und orange-korall wurden in der Herstellung chinesischen Schmucks und anderer Arten chinesischer Kunst seit Jahrzehnten verwandt. Opaleszenz ist eine Imitation des Halbedelsteins Opal. Licht schillert auf dieser Farbe wie auf einem Opal; es ist sogar feurig wie ein Opal. Die abgebildete, bunt schillernde Puderdose hat drei Musikinstrument-spielende Musen als Griff.

Wegen ihres wahren Kunstwertes begannen die tschechoslowakischen Parfümflaschen und Accessoires in den

letzten Jahren an Beachtung und Schätzung zu gewinnen. Sie wurden umsichtig entworfen und sorgfältig gearbeitet, wie mit den Flaschen dieses Artikels bewiesen ist und besonders bei denen des gleichen Stils, aber verschiedener Farben. Die in drei Farben gezeigte Flasche, rot-korall, lapis- und malachitfarben, verkörpert Leda, die mythologische Figur "Leda und der Schwan". Sie demonstriert mehrere Fakten. Erstens: Die Flaschen wurden alle einzeln handgefertigt, nicht auf einem Fliessband massenproduziert. Alle drei Ledas sind etwas verschieden in ihrer Grösse, und diese Variante besteht nicht nur in der Gesamthöhe der Flaschen, sondern sie unterscheiden sich auch in jedem anderen Punkt, vom Boden bis zum Rand. sie variieren in der Grösse zwischen 6 1/4 und 6 1/2 inches. Weil die Stöpsel wahrscheinlich alle mit der Schmirgel-Methode handgefertigt wurden, können sie nicht ausgewechselt werden. Zweitens: Opak-Farben wurden nicht immer mit den passenden Opak-Stöpseln gepaart; einige wurden mit durchsichtigen gemacht, die extra entworfen wurden. Bei diesen drei Flaschen handelt es sich um perfekte Beispiele, dies zu bestätigen. Der Entwurf der Blumen auf den Stöpseln der roten und grünen Flaschen dupliziert vollkommen den Blumen-Entwurf, der sich entlang der Seiten der Flaschen befindet. Es ist offensichtlich, dass die Kombination richtig ist. Drittens: Diese Flaschen wurden sorgfältig entworfen. Gezeigt ist eine Original-Blaupause dieser Flasche, die erst kürzlich entdeckt und gerettet werden konnte, da sie fast für immer in einem Feuer verlorengegangen wäre. Da die Flasche nur eine wunderschöne Aktfigur zeigt, wäre es eine Spekulation, sie Leda zu nennen. Jedoch zeigt die passende Puderdose klar und deutlich, dass es sich wirklich um Leda handelt, da sich die Erscheinung des Schwans auf dem Deckel der Puderdose befindet. Viertens: Die Original-Blaupause zeigt, dass Stöpsel und Flasche individuell entworfen und dann zusammengefügt wurden und eine Design-Kombinations-Nr. vergeben wurde. Für die Leda-Flasche, die in drei Farben gezeigt wird, war die Design-Nr. für die Flasche 513, für den Stöpsel 621. Die Kombinations-Nr. für diese beiden war die Design-Nr. 52678. Die passende Puderdose zeigt, dass die Dose selbst die Nr. 565 hat, der Deckel die Nr. 566 und die Kombination der beiden die Nr. 1079. Fünftens: Wie die Blaupause ebenfalls beweist, ist der gezeigte Stöpsel nicht der gleiche Entwurf wie die Stöpsel der drei Beispiele. In vielen Fällen haben die Schöpfer der tschechischen Parfümflaschen mehr als einen Stöpsel für jede Basis und umgekehrt entworfen.

Obwohl Kunsterzeugnisse aus Glas heutzutage zweifellos in mehreren Teilen der Welt entworfen und gefertigt werden, erreichte die von den Böhmen demonstrierte einmalige Kunstfertigkeit ihren Zenit in Form tschechoslowakischer Parfümflaschen während der zwei Dekaden zwischen den zwei Weltkriegen dieses Jahrhunderts. Diese kurze Periode der Geschichte erzeugte Schätze, die mit jedem vorübergehenden Tag von mehr und mehr Sammlern geschätzt werden.

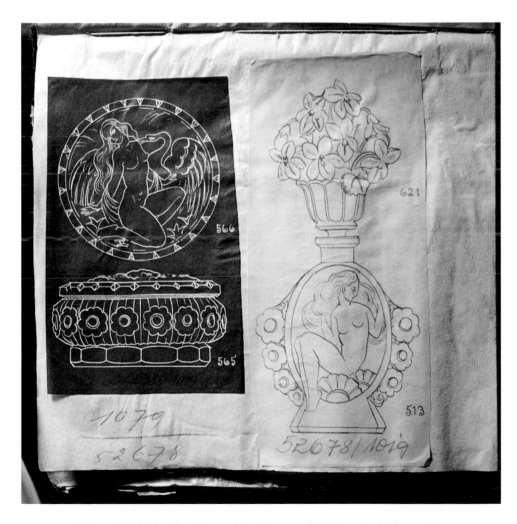

Figure 17. Original Czech artwork for the perfume bottles seen in Figure 16.
Collection of Donna Sims.

Rue de la Paix - Place Vendôme

| From 1840 to 1940: Crucible of the French Perfume Industry for a Century | de 1840 à 1940: Écrin et Creuset d'un Siècle de Grande Parfumerie Française |

Jean Blanchard

From the middle of the 19th century until the middle of the 20th century (when decentralisation of the perfume industry took place), an extremely well-defined geographic location represented by the Rue de la Paix and the Place Vendôme was truly the world dissemination center for the luxury perfume industry not only within France but throughout the world. If one enlarges the zone to the streets surrounding the Rue de la Paix (Rue des Capucines, Place de L'Opéra) and to the Rue du Faubourg St. Honoré (which lets out onto the Place Vendôme) and its continuation the Rue St. Honoré, this area includes almost all the perfume houses which took root there during the time from 1840 to 1950.

A brief sketch of the history of this locale is appropriate. Before it became a center of luxury and elegance with the stores of the great fashion designers, perfume houses, and jewellers, the area of the Place Vendôme and the Rue de la Paix underwent numerous modifications. It was at the initiative of Louvois, in the years 1670-1680, that the Place Vendôme was first created, at the site of the Vendôme Mansion, giving rise to the creation of a hexagonal area with facets cut at every angle. Between 1696 and 1728, under the reign of Louis XIV and then under Louis XV, the construction of this Place Vendôme saw Louvois succeded by Hardouin, and then Mansard and Boffrard. The greatest architects of the era thus each participated in the elaboration of this architectural jewel of the late 17th century. The Rue de la Paix was cut through in 1806 on the site

A l'échelle parisienne, et plus encore internationale, durant plus d'un siècle, soit entre le milieu du XIXème siècle, jusqu'au milieu de XXème siècle qui verra la diversification et la décentralisation des sites de présentation de la parfumerie de luxe, une entité géographique extrêmement limitée, représentée par la rue de la Paix et la Place Vendôme, fut réellement le centre mondial de rayonnement de la grande parfumerie de luxe tant française, pour une grande part, qu'internationale. Si l'on élargi la zone aux rues adjacentes de la Rue de la Paix (Rue des Capucines, Place de L'Opéra) et à la rue du Faubourg St. Honoré (qui débouche sur la Place Vendôme) et sa continuation la rue St. Honoré, c'est la quasi totalité des marques de parfumerie qui s'implantèrent là, au cours du siècle et un peu plus s'écoulant entre les années 1840 et 1950.

Il convient de rappeler par un bref aperçu l'histoire de ces lieux. Avant d'être un haut-lieu de l'élégance et du luxe, où se concentrèrent les ateliers et les magasins de vente des grands couturiers, parfumeurs et joailliers, le quartier de la Place Vendôme et de la Rue de la Paix connût diverses modifications. C'est à l'initiative de Louvois, dans les années 1670-1680 que la Place Vendôme fut créée, à l'emplacement de l'Hôtel de Vendôme, qui décida la création d'une place hexagonale à pans coupés à chaque angle. Entre 1686 et 1728, sous le règne de Louis XIV puis Louis XV, la construction de longue haleine de cette place vit se succèder le même Louvois, puis Hardouin, et enfin Mansart

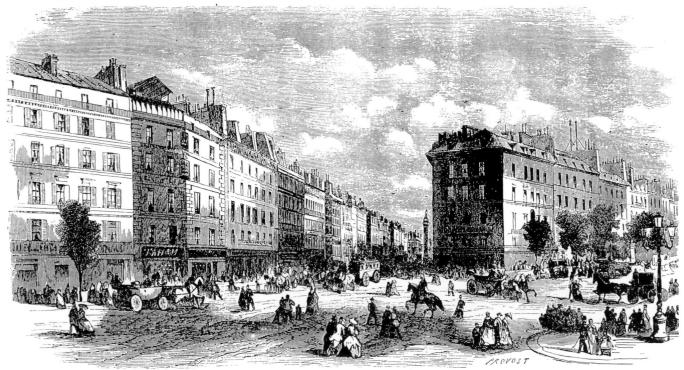

LES DÉMOLITIONS A PARIS. — Aspect de l'entrée de la rue de la Paix avant le percement de la rue de l'Impératrice. — D'après un croquis de M. Pignard.

Figure 1. A view of the entrance of the Rue de la Paix before the building of the rue de l'Imperatrice.

of the former convent of the Capucines, and initially bore the name Rue Napoléon (who then reigned at the height of his European conquests) and was given its present name ['Street of Peace'] after 1814, referring to the peace treaty of 1814 and bearing a less imperialist message.

It should be noted that the Place Vendôme was gaslit beginning in 1828, a little before the Rue de la Paix, which reminds the perfume bottle collector of the Corday *Rue de la Paix*, representing a streetlamp of green metal, an exact replica of the 19th century streetlamps which lit Paris from 1817 from the Passage du Panorama to the Palais Royal. Later, in the second half of the 19th century, the appearance of the Rue de la Paix was altered because of the restructuring work in Paris of Baron Haussmann, who did away with a good number of dark, narrow streets and replaced them with wide streets lined with buildings made of sculpted stone, called "Haussmanns." The great perfume houses did not take root here in isolation, but rather concomitantly with those of high fashion (often associated, but especially after the beginning of the 20th century) and of fine jewelry; the great names of contemporary jewelry had also colonized the most prestigious addresses on the Place Vendôme, but some among them, such as Chaumet, had been firmly planted there for more than two centuries.

Paradoxically, it was a great perfume house, perhaps the greatest, not only in reputation but also in commercial success, which for independent reasons of its own put a stop to the conforming character of business on the Rue de la Paix - Place Vendôme. In effect, it was Guerlain, founded in 1828 at 42, Rue de Rivoli by Pierre François Pascal Guerlain, which more or less initiated the success of the Rue de la Paix in 1840 by moving its store there, and contributed greatly to the installation of other perfumeries who had witnessed the success of the Guerlain store at 15, Rue de la Paix. Its fame was established firmly after 1853, when

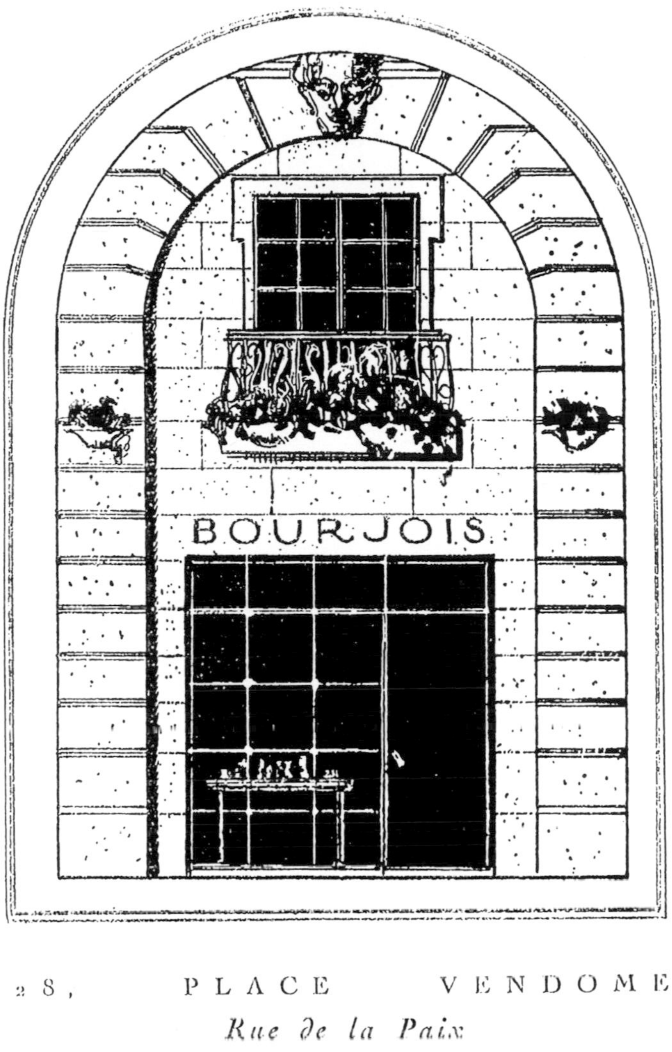

28, PLACE VENDOME
Rue de la Paix

Figure 2. An advertisement by Bourjois, showing its location at 28, Place Vendôme, (Rue de la Paix).

et Boffrard. Les plus grands architectes de l'époque participèrent donc à l'élaboration de ce joyau de l'architecture fin XVIIème-début XVIIIème. La Rue de la Paix, quant à elle, fut percée en 1806 sur l'emplacement de l'ancien couvent des Capucines, initialement sous le nom de Rue Napoléon (qui règnait alors, au faîte de ses conquêtes européennes), remplacé à partir du 1814 par le nom actuel s'appliquant au traité de paix de 1814, et porteur d'un message politique moins impérialiste.

Il faut noter que la Place Vendôme fut éclairée au gaz dès 1828, peu avant la Rue de la Paix, ce qui évoque chez les collectionneurs de flacons à parfum la réminiscence du flacon de Corday *Rue de la Paix*, représentant un réverbère en régule vert, exact réplique des réverbères à gaz du 19ème siècle, qui éclairèrent Paris dès 1817, au Passage du Panorama au Palais Royal. Plus tardivement, dans la seconde moitié du XIXème siècle, l'aspect de la Rue de la Paix changea au moment des travaux de restructuration de Paris du Baron Haussmann (qui fit disparaître bon nombre de rues étroites et insalubres par des rues larges et bordées d'immeubles en pierre de taille, dits haussmaniens). Comme je l'évoquais, l'implantation des grandes marques de parfumerie ne se fit pas isolément, mais de façon concomitante avec celle de la couture (souvent associées dans un complémentarité entre couture et parfum, mais ce surtout à partir du début du XXème siècle), et de la haute joaillerie (les grands noms de la joaillerie contemporaine ont colonisés les adresses les plus prestigieuses de la Place Vendôme, mais certaines d'entre-elles comme Chaumet sont implantées là depuis plus de deux siècles).

Paradoxalement, c'est un grand parfumeur, peut-être le plus grand, tant en notoriété qu'en réussite commerciale, qui pour des raisons indépendantes de sa volonté sonna le glas du caractère incontournable de

Guerlain had become the official perfumer to the Empress Eugénie (especially for the *Eau de Cologne Impériale*) and then also to numerous royal houses of Europe.

The dynamism and vitality of the Guerlain enterprise encouraged the installation of other perfumers there, such as Rigaud in 1854 and Bourjois in 1860. The uprooting of the Guerlain store was provoked by the fact that a little before the start of the First World War, in 1914, the Doucet family, a house of high fashion (and in 1929 also of perfume), refused to renew Guerlain's lease, after a tenancy of almost 75 years. The Guerlain heirs were forced to find a new location to continue their business. They chose the Champs-Elysées, in a golden triangle of modern buildings, but this once again represented a risk because of the decentralized nature of the location, and especially at a time when the Champs-Elysées, before the war of 1914-1918, represented a place for Sunday strolls, almost as if in the country. Their moving was not a smooth one, because Guerlain publicly denounced their landlord's betrayal in *Le Figaro* and also in certain American newspapers, and they took their time at freeing up the location by waiting until the very last year of the lease, 1923. But all collectors will always remember the perfume *Rue de la Paix*, created by Guerlain in 1908, with its label decorated with a picture of the store at 15, Rue de la Paix, from the angle of the Rue des Capucines, and with the Vendôme Column in the background.

The Worth company was created in Paris in 1858, three years after Charles Frédéric Worth, of English nationality, landed there with 117 francs in his pocket and speaking not a word of French. In 1858 he joined with a Swede, Bobérg, and with a man of Dutch nationality and founded a fashion establishment at 7, Rue de la Paix, not far from Paquin. Their success was immediate, because of the new tone they brought to feminine fashion. But it was not until 1924 that his son Philippe created Parfums Worth, of which the perfume bottles designed by René

l'implantation Rue de la Paix - Place Vendôme. En effet, Guerlain, qui initia quasiment le succès de la Rue de la Paix en 1840, en déménageant ses locaux (inauguraux) fondés en 1828 au 42, rue de Rivoli par Pierre François Pascal Guerlain, contribua grandement à l'implantation d'autres parfumeurs qui voyaient la réussite de la Boutique Guerlain du 15 Rue de la Paix. La notoriété s'établit véritablement à partir de 1853, date à laquelle la maison Guerlain devint fournisseur officiel de l'Imperatrice Eugénie (en particulier pour l'Eau de Cologne Impériale), puis d'une multitude de cours royales d'Europe.

Le dynamisme et la multiplicité des productions de la maison Guerlain favorisent l'installation de maisons telles que Rigaud en 1854, puis Bourjois en 1860. Le déménagement de Guerlain fut provoqué par le fait que peu avant le début de la Grande Guerre, en 1914, la famille Doucet, elle-même implantée dans la couture, puis en 1929 dans la parfumerie, refusa le renouvellement du bail, après près de 75 ans de location des locaux. Les héritiers Guerlain se virent imposer de trouver un lieu de remplacement pour continuer leurs activités. Ils choisirent les Champs-Elysées, dans le triangle d'Or de l'immobilier moderne, mais qui, une fois de plus représentait un risque, compte tenu du caractère décentralisé du lieu, à une époque où les Champs Elysées, avant la guerre de 1914-1918, représentait surtout le lieu de promenade dominicale, quasiment à la campagne.

Cette réimplantation se fit non sans heurts, puisque Guerlain dénonça publiquement dans le Figaro ainsi que dans certains journaux américains, la traîtrise de son bailleur, et fit preuve de lenteur dans l'application des conditions de libération des locaux en allant jusqu'au bout des 9 ans du dernier bail échu, soit jusqu'en 1923. Mais tous les collectionneurs garderont à jamais en mémoire le souvenir de *Rue de la Paix*, parfum créé par Guerllain en 1908, à l'étiquette décorée

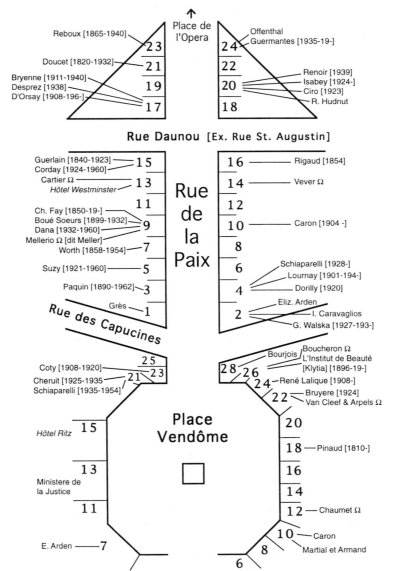

Figure 3. A map of the area of the Place Vendôme and Rue de la Paix, showing the locations of the Perfume Companies, Jewelers [marked with Ω], and Couturiers.

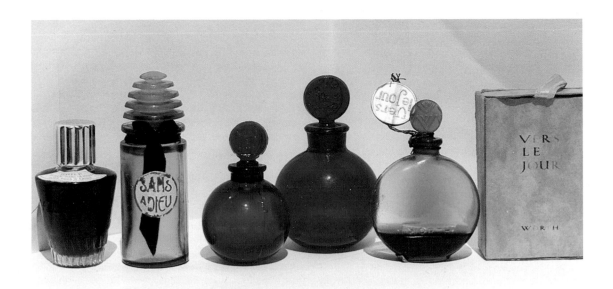

Figure 4. Perfume Miniatures of the house of Worth, located at 7, Rue de la Paix. Collection of Jean Blanchard.

Lalique are still a landmark achievement for both commercial and artistic success.

The Bourjois establishment, created in 1840 by Alexandre Napoléon Bourjois, was originally a manufacturer of theater make-up; they moved to 28 Place Vendôme in 1860 and soon became a famous perfumer, with their perfume *Manon Lescaut* of 1890. The Wertheimer family took over the Bourjois company and developed the marketing of their perfumes in Europe and in the United States for over fifty years (*Ashes of Roses, Evening in Paris*).

The d'Orsay company was created in 1908 by Mr. Van Dyck, a French citizen of Dutch origin, and by a German; they chose a location at 17, Rue de la Paix, which was by then already a center of luxury, and a castle for their office, complete with the name and coat of arms of an aristocrat from the 1830's, the Count d'Orsay, all this to give the image of luxury to their products, which were priced nonetheless in the moderate range. Their success was complete; in 1933, they sold over five million bottles of *Eau de Cologne d'Orsay*. Fortunately, many of their luxury perfume presentations are esthetically enchanting, due to the collaboration with René Lalique. In addition, some of their (replica) miniatures, though more recent, are singular achievements in quality and rarity (*Divine, Fantastique, Intoxication,* the shell bottle for *Le Dandy*).

Much later, in 1927, Elsa Schiaparelli opened a fashion boutique at 4, Rue de la Paix, and moved to 21, Place Vendôme after the enterprise expanded to include perfumes. The originality and high quality of her creations are cherished by all collectors of perfume bottles and of high fashion. Her Lobster Dress, the color Shocking Pink, the dress dummy shape of the perfume *Shocking,* the woman's torso cut at the waist and with her skirt fallen to the ankles for the perfume *Zut,* the candle for *Shocking,* the fig leaf for *Succès Fou,* the bottle of Chianti for *Si,* the sunburst face of *Le Roy Soleil* are imbued with a surrealist influence and an extreme creativity combined with rarity for many of her creations.

To complete their international renown and commercial success, two great American perfume companies

d'une vue du Magasin du 15, à l'angle de la Rue des Capucines, avec la Colonne Vendôme au 2ème plan.

La maison Worth, elle, est créée à Paris en 1858, trois ans après que Charles Frédéric Worth, de nationalité anglaise, ait débarqué avec 117 francs en poche et ne parlant pas un mot de français. En 1858, il s'associe au Suèdois Bobérg et à un autre associé Néerlandais et fonde une boutique de couture au 7, Rue de la Paix, non loin de Paquin. Le succès est immédiat grâce au ton nouveau insufflé à la mode féminine, mais c'est seulement en 1924 que son fils Philippe crée les Parfums Worth, dont les flacons créés par René Lalique restent des références de réussite à la fois artistique et commerciale.

La maison Bourjois, créée en 1840 par Alexandre Napoléon Bourjois, et initialement fabricant de fards de théâtre, s'implante au 28 de la Place Vendôme en 1860, et devient rapidement un parfumeur renommé, avec le parfum *Manon Lescaut* en 1890. La famille Wortheimer reprend les rênes de la maison Bourjois et développe à l'échelle Européenne, puis Américaine la diffusion de ses parfums pendant près de 50 ans (*Ashes of Roses, Evening in Paris*).

La Societé d'Orsay, créée en 1908 par M. Van Dyck, néerlandais naturalisé français et un associé allemand, fit le choix d'une implantation au 17 Rue de la Paix, alors le centre du luxe, d'un siège social dans un château et du nom et des armoiries d'un aristocrate des années 1830, le comte d'Orsay, pour donner l'image du luxe, mais à prix moyens. La réussite fut totale puisqu'en 1933, 5 millions de flacons de Eau de Cologne d'Orsay furent vendus. Heureusement, quelques présentations de grand luxe dûes à la collaboration avec René Lalique représentent de réels enchantements esthétiques. De même certaines miniatures plus récentes, et souvent répliques, sont des références dans la qualité et la rareté (*Divine, Fantastique, Intoxication,* flacon coquillage pour *Le Dandy*).

Beaucoup plus tardivement, Elsa Schiaparelli ouvre, en 1927, une boutique de couture au 4 de la Rue de la Paix, et déménage à quelques pas de là, au 21 de la Place Vendôme un an après avoir diversifié sa production aux parfums. L'originalité et la haute qualité de sa produc-

opened luxurious stores on Rue de la Paix, separate but at the same number 20, in 1923 for Ciro and in 1927 for Richard Hudnut. The luxurious interior decor of the Richard Hudnut store is the best known, and represents a focal achievement of the luxuries of the Art Deco era. Actually, the stores at 20, Rue de la Paix (which were featured on black and white post cards of the time) combined furniture, interior design, and merchandise all of high quality which flaunted their elitist character. The quintessence of luxury of Richard Hudnut was the famous bottle *Le Début* which was created in 1927 and was produced in four fragrances each with a different color.

The fashion designers such as the Soeurs Boué or Isabelle Caravaglios, established respectively at 9, and at 2, Rue de la Paix since the turn of the 20th century, also produced lines of high quality perfume, but with irregular success; avid collectors today hunt them actively since they were distributed in a very limited manner. These complete the palette of the luxury industries which were then at the disposition of the elegant public in this very limited geographic area.

On the other hand, some perfume companies, whether related or not to the fashion industry, declined to have stores in this narrow perimeter. In some cases, because the strong personality of their directors (cf. Gabrielle Chanel) which allowed them to be sure that the quality of their product would guarantee significant commercial success. Of course Chanel did not start making perfumes until after 1921. In some cases because the cost of renting space in this quarter became prohibitive by the end of the 19th century (cf. the example of Guerlain). Or finally, because many perfume companies arrived upon the commercial scene after the peak in the popularity of this area. Two chronologically comparable examples are Christian Dior and Nina Ricci, perfume companies founded after the Second World War, both originally houses of *haute couture*, which did not use locations on the Rue de la Paix/ Place Vendôme and which developed an opposite attraction pole for fashion and perfume of the post-war era. And it was indeed this which attracted Caron toward the Avenue Montaigne, which had been at 10, Rue de la Paix and then at 10 Place Vendôme from 1903 to 1950.

To return to Chanel, at the time of the renewal of the Place Vendôme-Rue de la Paix begun in the 1960's but which is still ongoing (initiated by the great international houses of jewelry), this famous house founded on the Rue Cambon finally opened a boutique devoted to fine jewelry on the Place Vendôme in 1990. But Mlle. Gabrielle Chanel had passed away twenty years before—she who had spent a great part of her life at the Hotel Ritz, fifty yards from there, located on the Place Vendôme. The circle had been made complete.

tion tant dans le domaine de la haute couture que de la grande parfumerie restent emblématiques pour tous les amateurs d'habillement ou de fragrances. La Robe Homard, les couleurs Rose Shocking et les formes de flacon buste de couturière pour le parfum *Shocking*, de corps de femme coupé aux hanches, en sous vêtements, la jupe tombée aux chevilles pour *Zut*, de Chandelier pour *Sleeping*, de feuille de vigne pour *Succès Fou*, de bouteille de chianti pour *Si*, de soleil rayonnant pour *Le Roy Soleil* resteront empreintes d'une influence surréaliste et d'une créativité extrême, associées à une rareté pour de nombreuses créations.

Pour parfaire leur renommée internationale et leur réussite commerciale deux grands parfumeurs américains ouvriront de luxueuses boutiques Rue de la Paix, distinctes mais au même No. 20, en 1923 pour Ciro et 1927 pour Richard Hudnut. L'aménagement intèrieur et le luxe de la boutique Richard Hudnut sont les mieux connus, et constituent une référence dans le domaine de luxe de des folies Art Déco. En effet, les salons de 20, Rue de la Paix (qui furent l'objet de photographies éditées en cartes postales sépia) combinaient un mobilier, une architecture intérieure et des marchandises de grande qualité, tout en affichant leur caractère élitiste. Dans le fameux flacon *Le Début* créé en 1927 et décliné en quatre fragrances de différentes couleurs, on retrouve la quintessence du luxe des productions Hudnut.

Les modistes comme les Soeurs Boué ou Isabelle Caravaglios, implantées respectivement au 9 et au 2 Rue de la Paix dès le tournant du XXème siècle, développèrent des gammes de parfumerie de qualité, au succès inconstant, mais que les grands collectionneurs actuels recherchent activement, car ayant fait l'objet d'une diffusion limitée, voire confidentielle. Elles complêtaient la palette des industries de luxe à la disposition des élégantes de l'époque dans un cadre géographique hyperconcentré.

A l'opposé, certaines maisons de parfumeries issues ou non de la couture, refusèrent de s'installer dans cet étroit périmètre:
•soit, parce que la forte personnalité de ses dirigeants (on pense à Gabrielle Chanel), lui permettait d'être sûre que la qualité de ses produits suffirait à lui assurer un succès commercial significatif.

•soit, parce que le coût des implantations dans ce quartier, prohibitif dès la fin de XIXème siècle (l'exemple Guerlain vient le corroborer) constituait un frein à cette localisation.

•soit enfin, pour des maisons arrivées plus tardivement sur le marché de la parfumerie au moment du déclin, ou en tout cas de la défervescence de la notoriété des lieux. En prenant deux exemples chronologiquement comparables, les maisons Christian Dior et Nina Ricci, parfumeurs après la seconde guerre mondiale, venues toutes deux de la couture n'envisagèrent pas de localisations Rue de la Paix - Place Vendôme et développèrent ainsi un autre pôle d'attraction du luxe Haute Couture - Parfumerie dès l'immédiat après guerre. Et c'est ceux-là même qui influenceront et "attireront" en 1950 les parfums Caron vers l'Avenue Montaigne, pourtant installés au 10 rue de la Paix, puis au 10 Place Vendôme de 1903 à 1950.

Pour en revenir à Chanel, au moment du renouveau de la Place Vendôme-Rue de la Paix, par l'entremise des grandes maisons de joaillerie internationales, dès les années 60 mais selon un processus encore actuel, la maison de la rue Cambon, implanta finalement en 1990 une boutique dévolue à la bijouterie de grand luxe, Place Vendôme. Mais Mlle. Gabrielle Chanel s'était éteinte depuis près de 20 ans, elle qui passa une grande partie de sa vie à l'Hotel Ritz, à 50 m de là, toujours Place Vendôme. La boucle était bouclée.

Correspondance for the author can be addressed to:
Jean Blanchard, 54, rue de Mortillet, 38000 Grenoble, France.

Rue de la Paix - Place Vendôme von 1840 bis 1940
Schmelztiegel der französischen Parfüm-Industrie für ein Jahrhundert

Von der Mitte des 19. bis zur Mitte des 20. Jahrhunderts (als die Dezentralisation der Parfüm-Industrie stattfand) war eine äusserst genau umgrenzbare Gegend, verkörpert durch die Rue de la Paix und den Place Vendôme, das Ausbreitungszentrum der luxuriösen Parfüm-Industrie nicht nur innerhalb Frankreichs sondern für die ganze Welt. Wenn man die Zone auf die umgebenden Strassen der Rue de la Paix (Rue des Capucines, Place de l'Opéra) und auf die Rue du Faubourg St. Honoré (die auf den Place Vendôme und seine Fortsetzung, die Rue St. Honoré mündet) erweitert, schliesst diese Gegend fast alle der Parfümhäuser ein, die dort während der Zeit von 1840 bis 1950 ihren Ursprung hatten.

Eine kurze Studie der Geschichte dieses Schauplatzes erweist sich als angemessen. Bevor sie ein Zentrum des Luxus und der Eleganz mit Läden der grossen Modeschöpfer, Parfümhäuser und Juweliere wurde, erlebte die Gegend des Place Vendômes und der Rue de la Paix zahlreiche Veränderungen. In den Jahren 1670 bis 1680 wurde der Place Vendôme auf der Stelle des Herrenhauses Vendôme, aufgrund der Initiative von Louvois, ins Leben gerufen und liess ein in jedem Winkel facettenreich gestaltetes sechseckiges Gebiet entstehen. Zwischen 1696 und 1728, unter der Herrschaft von Louis XIV und dann Louis XV, folgten in der Gestaltung dieses Place Vendôme nach Louvois erst Hardouin und später Mansard und Boffrard. Die grössten Architekten dieser Ära nahmen somit an der Ausführung dieses architektonischen Juwels des späten 17. Jahrhunderts teil. Die Rue de la Paix wurde in 1806 an der Stelle des ehemaligen Kapuziner-Klosters geteilt, und hatte ursprünglich den Namen Rue Napoléon (der auf der Höhe seiner europäischen Eroberung herrührte) und erhielt ihren derzeitigen Namen ("Strasse des Friedens") nach 1814, bezugnehmend auf das Friedensabkommen von 1814, und trug somit eine weniger imperialistische Botschaft.

Es sollte erwähnt werden, dass der Place Vendôme mit Beginn des Jahres 1828 mit Gaslaternen beleuchtet wurde, etwas früher als die Rue de la Paix, was den Parfümflaschen-Sammler an Corday's Rue de la Paix erinnert, welches eine grün-metallene Strassenlaterne darstellt, eine genaue Wiedergabe der Strassenlaternen des 19. Jahrhunderts, die Paris von der Passage du Panorame bis zum Palais Royal von 1817 an erhellten. Später, in der zweiten Hälfte des 19. Jahrhunderts, wurde das Erscheinungsbild der Rue de la Paix aufgrund der Umbauarbeiten in Paris durch Baron Haussmann verändert, der eine grosse Zahl von dunklen, engen Strassen mit breiten Strassen ersetzte, mit Häusern in bildhauerischem Baustil, genannt "Haussmanns". Die Gründungen der grossen Parfümhäuser fanden hier keineswegs isoliert statt, sondern in Begleitung mit den Häusern der eleganten Mode (oftmals zusammengeschlossen, jedoch besonders nach dem Beginn des 20. Jahrhunderts) und denen des edlen Schmucks. Die grossen Namen des zeitgenössischen Schmucks hatten ebenfalls die angesehensten Adressen auf dem Place Vendôme eingenommen, jedoch waren einige unter ihnen hier schon für über zwei Jahrzehnte fest angesiedelt, wie z.B. Chaumet.

Paradoxerweise war es ein grosses Parfümhaus, vielleicht sogar das grösste, nicht nur in seinem Ruf sondern auch in seinem kommerziellen Erfolg, welches aus unabhängigen eigenen Gründen dem gleichförmigen Charakter des Geschäftslebens auf der Rue de la Paix - Place Vendôme einen Einhalt gewährte. Tatsächlich war es Guerlain, in 1828 von Pierre Francois Pascal Guerlain auf der Rue de Rivoli No. 42 gegründet, der in 1840 mehr oder weniger den Erfolg der Rue de la Paix in Gang setzte, indem er sein Geschäft dorthin verlegte und so in starker Weise dazu beitrug, dass andere Parfümerien dort eingerichtet wurden, welche Zeugen des Erfolgs des Guerlain-Ladens auf der Rue de la Paix No. 15 waren. Sein Ruhm wurde nach 1853 fest etabliert, nachdem Guerlain der offizielle Parfumeur der Kaiserin Eugenie (besonders für das "Eau de Cologne Impériale") und dann auch von zahlreichen europäischen Königshäusern wurde.

Der Dynamismus und die Vitalität des Guerlain Unternehmens ermutigte dort die Einrichtung anderer Parfümerien,

wie Rigaud in 1854 und Bourjois in 1860. Die Entwurzlung des Guerlain Ladens wurde durch den Umstand provoziert, dass sich die Doucet-Familie (ein Haus eleganter Mode und in 1929 auch von Parfüm) in 1914, kurz vor dem Beginn des ersten Weltkriegs, weigerte - nach einer Dauer von fast 75 Jahren - Guerlain's Mietvertrag zu erneuern. Die Erben Guerlain's waren gezwungen, einen neuen Standort zu finden, um ihre Geschäfte fortsetzen zu können. Sie wählten die Champs Elysées, in einem goldenen Dreieck moderner Gebäude, was jedoch, aufgrund der Dezentralisation des Standorts, wiederum ein Risiko bedeutete, besonders zu einer Zeit, als die Champs Elysées (vor dem Krieg von 1914-1918) einen Platz für Sonntagsspazierer darstellte, fast wie auf dem Lande. Der Umzug ging nicht glatt vonstatten, da Guerlain öffentlich in "Le Figaro", und auch in bestimmten amerikanischen Zeitungen, seine Vermieter des Treuebruchs bezichtigte und den Umzug bis 1923, dem allerletzten Jahr des Mietvertrages hinausschob. Dessenungeachtet werden sich alle Sammler immer an das Parfüm Rue de la Paix erinnern, von Guerlain in 1908 geschaffen. Sein Etikett ist mit einem Bild des Ladens der Rue de la Paix No. 15 dekoriert, gesehen aus einem Winkel der Rue des Capucines, mit der Vendôme-Säule im Hintergrund. 1858 wurde das Unternehmen Worth in Paris gegründet, drei Jahre nachdem der Engländer Charles Frédéric Worth dort mit 117 französischen Franken in der Tasche angekommen war und nicht ein Wort französisch sprach. Im gleichen Jahr vereinigte er sich mit einem Schweden, Bobérget, und mit einem Mann holländischer Nationalität und gründete ein Mode-Unternehmen auf der Rue de la Paix No. 7, nicht weit von Paquin. Aufgrund des neuen Stils, den sie in die Damenmode einbrachten, waren sie sofort erfolgreich. Jedoch dauerte es bis 1924, dass sein Sohn Philippe Worth Parfüme kreierte, von denen die von René Lalique entworfenen Parfüm-Flaschen immer noch einen Markstein der Vollendung sowohl für kommerziellen als auch künstlerischen Erfolg darstellen.

Das Bourjois Unternehmen, von Alexandre Napoléon Bourjois in 1840 gegründet, war ursprünglich ein Hersteller von Theater-Schminke. Es siedelte in 1860 auf den Place Vendôme No. 20 um und entwickelte sich zu einem berühmten Parfümeriehändler mit seinem Parfüm Manon Lescaut von 1890. Die Bourjois Firma wurde von der Familie Wertheimer übernommen, und diese machte die Vermarktung deren Parfüme in Europa und den Vereinigten Staaten von Amerika über fünfzig Jahre lang nutzbar (Ashes of Roses, Evening in Paris).

Das Unternehmen d'Orsay wurde von Mr. Van Dyck, einem französischen Bürger holländischer Herkunft, und einem Deutschen in 1908 gegründet. Sie wählten eine Niederlassung auf der Rue de la Paix No. 17, welche zu dieser Zeit schon ein Luxuszentrum war und somit ein Schloss für deren Geschäfte, komplett mit dem Namen und dem Wappenschild eines Aristokraten der Jahre um 1830, dem Grafen d'Orsay. All dies gab deren Produkte den Anschein von Luxus, obwohl sie trotzalledem in einer angemessenen Preislage rangierten. Es war ein vollkommener Erfolg. In 1933 wurden über fünf Millionen Flaschen von Eau de Cologne d'Orsay verkauft. Es ist ein Glücksfall, dass viele ihrer luxuriösen Parfüm Präsentationen aufgrund der Zusammenarbeit mit René Lalique ästhetisch bezaubernd sind. Hinzu kommt, dass einige ihrer Miniatur-Nachbildungen, obwohl mehr jüngeren Datums, einmalige Ausführungen in Qualität und Seltenheit darstellen (Divine, Fantastique, Intoxication, die Muschel-Flasche für Le Dandy).

Erst viel später, in 1927, eröffnete Elsa Schiaparelli eine Mode-Boutique auf der Rue de la Paix No. 4 und zog auf den Place Vendôme No. 21 um, nachdem das Unternehmen expandierte und Parfüme einschloss. Die Originalität und höchste Qualität ihrer Kreationen werden von allen Sammlern von Parfümflaschen und denen eleganter Mode hoch geschätzt. Ihr Hummer-Kleid, in schockierendem pink-rosa, die Kleiderpuppenform des Parfüms Shocking mit dem an der Taille gekappten Frauentorso, ihrem bis zu den Knöcheln reichenden Rock für das Parfüm Zut, die Kerze für Shocking, das Feigenblatt für Succès Fou, die Chianti-Flasche für

Si und das sonnenflammende Gesicht für *Le Roy Soleil* sind alle durchdrungen von einem surrealistischen Einfluss, der mit einer extremen Kreativität und einer Rarität für viele ihrer Kreationen kombiniert ist.

Um ihren internationalen Ruhm und kommerziellen Erfolg zu vervollständigen, eröffneten zwei grosse amerikanische Parfüm Firmen luxuriöse Geschäfte auf der Rue de la Paix, separat voneinander aber unter derselben No. 20: In 1923 für Ciro und in 1927 für Richard Hudnut. Das luxuriöse Interieur des Richard Hudnut Ladens ist das am besten bekannte und stellt eine fokale Ausführung des Überflusses der Art Deco Ära dar. Tatsächlich vereinigten die Geschäfte der Rue de la Paix No. 20 (die auf schwarz-weissen Postkarten dieser Zeit dargestellt wurden) Möbel, Inneneinrichtung und Waren, welche alle von höchster Qualität waren und ihren auserlesenen Charakter zur Schau stellten. Die Quintessenz des Luxus Richard Hudnut's war die berühmte Flasche für *Le Début*, das in 1927 entworfen und in vier Wohlgerüchen produziert wurde, von denen jeder eine anderen Farbe hatte.

Modeschöpfer, wie Soeurs Boue oder Isabelle Caravaglios, die sich jeweils auf der Rue de la Paix No. 9 und No. 2 nach der Wende des 20. Jahrhunderts etablierten, produzierten ebenfalls eine Reihe von hoch qualifizierten Parfümen, jedoch mit unregelmässigem Erfolg. Sie werden heute von begierigen Sammlern emsig aufgestöbert, da sie nur in einer sehr limitierten Auflage produziert wurden. - Somit war die Palette der Luxus Industrie vervollständigt, die dem eleganten Publikum in dieser sehr begrenzten Gegend zur Verfügung stand.

Auf der anderen Seite lehnten es einige Parfüm Firmen ab, Geschäfte in diesem engen Umkreis zu haben, egal ob sie mit der Mode–Industrie verwandt waren oder nicht. In einigen Fällen aufgrund der starken Persönlichkeit ihrer Direktoren (z.B. Gabrielle Chanel), welche es ihnen erlaubte sicher zu sein, dass ihnen die Qualität ihrer Produkte bedeutsamen kommerziellen Erfolg garantierte. In anderen Fällen, da es die untragbaren Kosten zum Ende des 19. Jahrhunderts verhinderten, Anmietung in diesem Quartier vorzunehmen (siehe das Beispiel von Guerlain). Oder letztendlich, weil viele Parfüm-Firmen auf der kommerziellen Szene erst nach dem Höhepunkt der Popularität dieser Gegend eingetroffen sind. Zwei chronologisch vergleichbare Beispiele sind Christian Dior und Nina Ricci; Parfüm-Firmen die nach dem zweiten Weltkrieg gegründet wurden, beide Abkömmlinge der Mode-Industrie, welche keinen Gebrauch von der Gegend der Rue de la Paix/Place Vendôme machten und einen entgegengesetzten Pol der Anziehungskraft für Mode und Parfüm der Nachkriegszeit entwickelten. Und in der Tat zog es Caron aus diesem Grund zur Avenue Montaigne hin, der sich von 1903 bis 1950 auf der Rue de la Paix No. 10 und dann auf dem Place Vendôme No. 10 befand.

Um zu Chanel zurückzukehren, in der Zeit als die Erneuerung des Place Vendôme - Rue de la Paix in den 60er Jahren begann und indessen immer noch weitergeht (in Gang gesetzt durch die grossen internationalen Juwelier-Häuser); eröffnete dieses berühmte Haus, das auf der Rue Cambon gegründet war, letztendlich in 1990 eine Boutique auf dem Place Vendôme, die dem edlen Schmuck gewidmet ist. Aber Mlle. Gabrielle Chanel war schon vor zwanzig Jahren dahingeschieden. —Sie, die einen grossen Teil ihres Lebens im Hotel Ritz verbracht hatte, knapp fünfzig Meter entfernt, auf dem Place Vendôme gelegen. Und somit hat sich der Kreis wieder geschlossen.

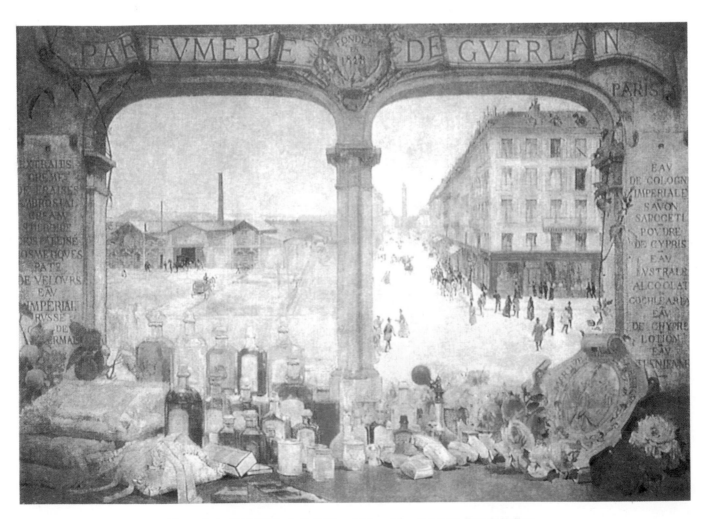

Figure 5. La Parfumerie de Guerlain, which was located at 15, Rue de la Paix.

MONSEN AND BAER

(703) 938-2129   BOX 529 Vienna, VA 22183   FAX: (703) 242-1357

ACTUAL PRICES REALIZED

Monsen and Baer Perfume Bottle Auction VI - May 11, 1996. San Francisco, California [Burlingame, CA].
The prices listed include the 10% buyer's commission.
Omitted lot numbers represent lots which were unsold or withdrawn as of the publication of this list.

LOT #	PRICE	LOT #	PRICE	LOT #	PRICE	LOT #	PRICE	LOT #	PRICE	LOT #	PRICE	LOT #	PRICE
1.	$132.00.	57.	$99.00.	113.	$143.00.	170.	$605.00.	226.	$55.00.	282.	$220.00.	346.	$264.00.
2.	$231.00.	58.	$132.00.	114.	$132.00.	171.	$231.00.	227.	$176.00.	283.	$165.00.	347.	$110.00.
3.	$605.00.	59.	$88.00.	115.	$66.00.	172.	$264.00.	228.	143.00.	284.	$1,320.00.	348.	$605.00.
4.	$110.00.	60.	$220.00.	116.	$44.00.	173.	$176.00.	229.	$319.00.	285.	$231.00.	349.	$319.00.
5.	$330.00.	61.	$242.00.	117.	$77.00.	174.	$154.00.	230.	$154.00.	286.	$33.00.	350.	$176.00.
6.	$231.00.	62.	$77.00.	118.	$220.00.	175.	$187.00.	231.	$66.00.	287.	$154.00.	351.	$143.00.
7.	$77.00.	63.	$88.00.	119.	$110.00.	176.	$412.50.	232.	$467.50.	288.	$110.00.	352.	$286.00.
8.	$286.00.	64.	$165.00.	120.	$330.00.	177.	$165.00.	233.	$66.00.	289.	$412.50.	353.	$165.00.
9.	$209.00.	65.	$77.00.	121.	$154.00.	178.	$660.00.	234.	$121.00.	290.	$143.00.	354.	$198.00.
10.	$209.00.	66.	$66.00.	122.	$330.00.	179.	$467.50.	235.	$88.00.	291.	$242.00.	355.	$550.00.
11.	$770.00.	67.	$99.00.	123.	$77.00.	180.	$88.00.	236.	$660.00.	292.	$308.00.	356.	$209.00.
12.	$275.00.	68.	$99.00.	124.	$110.00.	181.	$1,980.00.	237.	$121.00.	293.	$412.50.	357.	$209.00.
13.	$319.00.	69.	$154.00.	125.	$357.50.	182.	$357.50.	238.	$154.00.	294.	$308.00.	358.	$264.00.
14.	$1,430.00.	70.	$55.00.	126.	$467.50.	183.	$687.50.	239.	$165.00.	295.	$440.00.	359.	$143.00.
15.	$935.00.	71.	$88.00.	127.	$121.00.	184.	$522.50.	240.	$880.00.	206.	$231.00.	360.	$412.50.
16.	$660.00.	72.	$8,250.00.	128.	$198.00.	185.	$319.00.	241.	$88.00.	297.	$132.00.	361.	$231.00.
17.	$880.00.	73.	$220.00.	129.	$110.00.	186.	$77.00.	242.	$121.00.	298.	$495.00.	362.	$467.50.
18.	$22.00.	74.	$231.00.	130.	$220.00.	187.	$660.00.	243.	$77.00.	299.	$412.50.	363.	$522.50.
19.	$88.00.	75.	$467.50.	131.	$110.00.	188.	$198.00.	244.	$1,100.00.	300.	$440.00.	364.	$242.00.
20.	$231.00.	76.	$242.00.	132.	$242.00.	189.	$605.00.	245.	$231.00.	301.	$715.00.	365.	$198.00.
21.	$220.00.	77.	$1045.00.	133.	$1,650.00.	190.	$715.00.	246.	$110.00.	302.	$1,210.00.	366.	$165.00.
22.	$77.00.	78.	$231.00.	134.	$88.00.	191.	$132.00.	247.	$154.00.	303.	$1,210.00.	367.	$825.00.
23.	$385.00.	79.	$143.00.	135.	$143.00.	192.	$66.00.	248.	$385.00.	304.	$770.00.	368.	$357.50.
24.	$99.00.	80.	$231.00.	136.	$143.00.	193.	$357.50.	249.	$605.00.	305.	$1,870.00.	369.	$330.00.
25.	$165.00.	81.	$187.00.	137.	$143.00.	194.	$198.00.	250.	$88.00.	306.	$935.00.	370.	$357.50.
26.	$110.00.	82.	$286.00.	138.	$440.00.	195.	$198.00.	251.	$357.50.	307.	$5,225.00.	371.	$187.00.
27.	$187.00.	83.	$132.00.	139.	$198.00.	196.	$132.00.	252.	$550.00.	308.	$1,320.00.	372.	$357.50.
28.	$165.00.	84.	$242.00.	140.	$440.00.	197.	$715.00.	253.	$154.00.	309.	$2,750.00.	373.	$1,650.00.
29.	$467.50.	85.	$143.00.	141.	$286.00.	198.	$99.00.	254.	$357.50.	310.	$1,540.00.	374.	$550.00.
30.	$187.00.	86.	$357.50.	142.	$275.00.	199.	$231.00.	255.	$220.00.	311.	$2,200.00.	375.	$605.00.
31.	$264.00.	87.	$165.00.	143.	$275.00.	200.	$357.50.	256.	$357.50.	313.	$154.00.	376.	$110.00.
32.	$440.00.	88.	$330.00.	144.	$385.00.	201.	$88.00.	257.	$385.00.	315.	$198.00.	377.	$286.00.
33.	$176.00.	89.	$231.00.	145.	$198.00.	202.	$165.00.	258.	$253.00.	316.	$385.00.	378.	$1,320.00.
34.	$550.00.	90.	$165.00.	146.	$440.00.	203.	$132.00.	259.	$165.00.	317.	$1,045.00.	379.	$330.00.
35.	$44.00.	91.	$605.00.	147.	$357.50.	204.	$165.00.	260.	$286.00.	319.	$495.00.	380.	$1,320.00.
36.	$231.00.	92.	$66.00.	148.	$385.00.	205.	$55.00.	261.	$121.00.	320.	$209.00.	381.	$412.50.
37.	$176.00.	93.	$66.00.	149.	$330.00.	206.	$176.00.	262.	$412.50.	322.	$385.00.	382.	$1,540.00.
38.	$220.00.	94.	$154.00.	151.	$605.00.	207.	$187.00.	263.	$330.00.	323.	$357.50.	383.	$330.00.
39.	$88.00.	95.	$99.00.	152.	$1,210.00.	208.	$522.50.	264.	$231.00.	324.	$660.00.	384.	$412.50.
40.	$132.00.	96.	$286.00.	153.	$2,200.00.	209.	$660.00.	265.	$275.00.	325.	$935.00.	385.	$715.00.
41.	$66.00.	97.	$440.00.	154.	$66.00.	210.	$357.50.	266.	$275.00.	326.	$1,870.00.	386.	$357.50.
42.	$357.50.	98.	$412.50.	155.	$132.00.	211.	$715.00.	267.	$143.00.	329.	$220.00.	387.	$550.00.
43.	$88.00.	99.	$286.00.	156.	$143.00.	212.	$77.00.	268.	$825.00.	330.	$220.00.	388.	$605.00.
44.	$165.00.	100.	$66.00.	157.	$55.00.	213.	$132.00.	269.	$308.00.	331.	$132.00.	389.	$880.00.
45.	$55.00.	101.	$176.00.	158.	$121.00.	214.	$1,320.00.	270.	$143.00.	332.	$605.00.	390.	$2,970.00.
46.	$11.00.	102.	$88.00.	159.	$110.00.	215.	$143.00.	271.	$121.00.	333.	$440.00.	391.	$770.00.
47.	$99.00.	103.	$1,210.00.	160.	$176.00.	216.	$110.00.	272.	$264.00.	334.	$220.00.	392.	$880.00.
48.	$55.00.	104.	$110.00.	161.	$176.00.	217.	$176.00.	273.	$330.00.	335.	$308.00.	393.	$2,090.00.
49.	$77.00.	105.	$121.00.	162.	$176.00.	218.	$209.00.	274.	$825.00.	336.	$880.00.	394.	$1,210.00.
50.	$66.00.	106.	$143.00.	163.	$2,310.00.	219.	$330.00.	275.	$154.00.	338.	$1870.00.	395.	$2,860.00.
51.	$55.00.	107.	$110.00.	164.	$275.00.	220.	$187.00.	276.	$467.50.	340.	$9,350.00.		Want to be on
52.	$253.00.	108.	$220.00.	165.	$165.00.	221.	$412.50.	277.	$1,870.00.	341.	$110.00.		our Mailing List?
53.	$77.00.	109.	$88.00.	166.	$495.00.	222.	$77.00.	278.	$77.00.	342.	$330.00.		Just call or write.
54.	$220.00.	110.	$110.00.	167.	$935.00.	223.	$66.00.	279.	$110.00.	343.	$495.00.		Next Auction:
55.	$154.00.	111.	$110.00.	168.	$440.00.	224.	$110.00.	280.	$165.00.	344.	$440.00.		May 3, 1997
56.	$467.50.	112.	$121.00.	169.	$467.50.	225.	$990.00.	281.	$192.50.	345.	$253.00.		Washington, DC